BPPV
What You Need to Know

By P. J. Haybach, R.N., M.S.

Jerry L. Underwood, Ph.D., Editor

©2000 Vestibular Disorders Association

The Vestibular Disorders Association (VEDA) is a nonprofit organization that provides information and support to people with inner ear disorders. Founded in Portland, Oregon, in 1983, VEDA distributes information worldwide about the inner ear, the human balance system, benign paroxysmal positional vertigo (BPPV), Meniere's disease, labyrinthitis, and related topics through its many publications, its site on the World Wide Web of the Internet, and its quarterly newsletter, *On the Level.* Contact VEDA for more information or to become a member.

All rights reserved. No part of this book may be reprinted or reproduced or used in any form by any electronic, mechanical, or other means now known or hereinafter invented, included photocopying and recording, or in any information storage or retrieval system, without permission in writing from the Vestibular Disorders Association.

Printed in the United States of America.

Published by the Vestibular Disorders Association
PO Box 4467
Portland, OR 97208-4467
(800) 837-8428
veda@vestibular.org
http://www.vestibular.org

First Edition
Printed in the United States of America
10 9 8 7 6 5 4 3 2 1

International Standard Book Number: 0-9632611-3-4 (softcover)
0-9632611-4-2 (hardcover)

Table of Contents

Preface

We have written this book to fill the need for a basic work, understandable to the public, about benign paroxysmal positional vertigo (BPPV).

Our material is not limited to one viewpoint or approach. Instead, we have presented facts about BPPV, pros and cons about various treatments, and a wide variety of viewpoints expressed by other authors, researchers, health professionals, and people who have been diagnosed with BPPV.

We hope that our audience, after reading this book, will be well-informed about BPPV, its symptoms and signs, diagnostic testing, treatment options, coping strategies, and related issues. We also intend that our book be used to help educate family, friends, co-workers, employers, and others about the problem.

This book is not meant to substitute for professional health care or to promote or reject any particular theory or treatment.

BPPV: What You Need to Know is meant to enhance the doctor-patient relationship, not to replace it.

Dedication

BPPV: What You Need to Know is dedicated to the Haybach and Underwood families and to many good friends.

Acknowledgments

This book would not have been possible without the assistance of a great many people and organizations, including the medical and scientific advisors and the board of directors of the Vestibular Disorders Association.

The reference librarians of the Pinellas Park branch of the Pinellas County (Florida) Library were instrumental in obtaining many of the reference works needed to write this book.

Joyce Sherman, co-owner of River Graphics, Portland, Oregon, designed the book and coordinated indexing and printing.

The index was prepared by Monica Luce.

Chapter 1

Introduction

We have written this book mainly for people who have or suspect they have Benign Paroxysmal Positional Vertigo (BPPV) and want to know more about its nature, causes, diagnosis, and treatments as well as strategies for coping with its effects.

Here you'll find information about nearly every aspect of the disorder, from the basic anatomy and workings of the inner ear to things you should know about doctors, therapists, insurance companies, and support groups. We have also covered symptoms, the events thought to create symptoms, the tests, and the treatments. Along the way, we discuss research and how to learn more about libraries, associations, and the Internet.

The experience of BPPV varies from person to person. Not all the information in this book will apply to your particular case, but we hope this book will move you toward wise health-care decisions.

BPPV: What You Need To Know is not meant to substitute for discussions with your physician but to help you understand BPPV and to benefit more completely from your physician encounters. No book, including ours, can replace a knowledgeable and thorough physician who is familiar with BPPV and with your particular case.

What Is BPPV?

Benign paroxysmal positional vertigo is an inner-ear balance disorder characterized by sudden brief bouts of intense vertigo and nystagmus induced by specific head movements.

Definitions:
Benign: Not life-threatening, not progressive.
Paroxysmal: Occurring in sudden attacks.
Vertigo: Perception of movement (either of yourself or of objects around you) that is not occurring or is occurring differently from what you perceive.
Nystagmus: Abnormal jerking of the eyes that can be rotational or straight.
Positional vertigo: Vertigo caused by moving the head in a particular way (with respect to gravity).

Although BPPV is the most common vestibular problem, it is not fully understood, and complete agreement has not been reached about what it is (disease or set of symptoms), how to treat it, or what to call it.

Definition: The word **vestibular** can be used to refer to the balance function of the inner ear, the parts of the inner ear involved in balance, the structures involved in sending balance information to the brain, and the brain structure first receiving most of this information.

The Name

Several names are in use for BPPV. We have chosen the name "BPPV" for this condition because of its widespread use and to limit the chance for confusion. Other possible names for BPPV appear in Table 1-1.

Table 1-1: Other Names Sometimes Used for BPPV

Benign paroxysmal positional nystagmus (BPPN)
Benign positional vertigo
Paroxysmal positional nystagmus
Paroxysmal positional vertigo
Positional nystagmus of the benign paroxysmal type
Positional vertigo of the benign paroxysmal type

History

Barany described BPPV in the medical literature as early as 1921. In 1952, Dix and Hallpike described it again in English and referred to it as positional nystagmus of the benign paroxysmal type.

> "...the cause of the disease is essentially benign. It is seldom, if ever, we find, associated with any evidence of cranial disease (brain problems) and tends to recover with time and simple sedative measures. "

—Dix. M.R., and Hallpike, C.S., *Proceedings of the Royal Society of Medicine*, 1952.

> "The word benign is used to distinguish between types of vertigo caused by peripheral vestibular ailments and the type of vertigo caused by intracranial neoplasms. In fact, however, benign paroxysmal positional vertigo can be a severe disabling problem or a nagging nuisance responsible for constant frustration."

—J.M. Furman and S.P. Cass, *New England Journal of Medicine*, 1999.

A nurse with BPPV made the following comments about the word "benign" to describe this vestibular disorder:

> "BPPV is misnamed. The use of the word *benign* is deceptive. Its use leads the medical profession to treat the condition lightly. As well as meaning 'not malignant', benign means 'pleasant,' 'gentle,' 'favorable,' 'genial,' 'kind,' 'healthful' and 'beneficial.' Indeed, BPPV is quite the opposite. It is extremely unpleasant, extremely violent, extremely unfavorable, certainly unhealthy, and not beneficial in the slightest."
>
> —Mary B., RN, *More Stories and Strategies*, 1995

The paper by Dix and Hallpike also described a test for BPPV still extensively used today and known as the Dix-Hallpike maneuver.

Since 1952, many doctors have worked to learn more about what might occur within the inner ear to create the symptoms of BPPV. They have also worked on treatments, both medical and surgical. Medical treatment consisting of head movements was introduced in 1980, and other treatments have been added since. Although surgery is rarely needed to control vertigo, surgical procedures for BPPV have existed since the 1950s.

Statistics

Most experts regard BPPV as the most commonly diagnosed vestibular disorder. It accounts for at least 20 percent of diagnoses made by doctors specializing in dizziness and vestibular disorders. It is the most frequent cause of vertigo in the elderly. The number of people affected by this disorder each year has been estimated between 10 per 100,000 and 64 per 100,000 people, and some experts feel even more may be affected.

Using the Reference Sections

Most of the chapters in this book include a reference list of books and articles used in preparation of the chapter as well as others you might find interesting.

For journal citations, the names are those of the author or authors, if known. The article name appears in quotes. The title of the journal is italicized. The first number is the volume number (usually representing the number of years the journal has been published). The number, if any, in parentheses is the issue number (often representing the number of the month). The next numbers are the pages in the journal where you can find the article, and the last number is the year of publication.

For books, the names are those of the author or authors (if known). The book title appears in italics; then comes the city of publication, the publishing company's name, and the date of publication.

Disclaimer

The information in this book is not intended as a substitute for professional health care. Before acting on information found in this book, you should discuss it with your personal physician.

We have attempted to provide information about as many theories of the disease and treatments as possible to provide the fullest coverage of this disorder. We do not seek to impose our view of the "best" information or treatment, if indeed a best exists. Neither VEDA nor the author advocates any particular treatment for any particular disorder.

References

B., Mary. "Liberatory Maneuver." *More Stories and Strategies: Coping with Vestibular Disorders*. Portland, Ore.: Vestibular Disorders Association, 1995.

Baloh, R.W. *Dizziness, Hearing Loss, and Tinnitus*. Philadelphia: F.A. Davis Company, 1998.

Brookler, K.H., and Rubin, W. "Letter to the Editor", *Vestibular Update*, 9-4, Summer 1992.

Brandt, T. "Positional and Positioning Vertigo and Nystagmus." *Journal of the Neurological Sciences*, 95:2-28, 1990.

Dix, M.R., and Hallpike, C.S. "The Pathology, Symptomatology, and Diagnosis of Certain Common Disorders of the Vestibular System." *Proceedings of the Royal Society of Medicine*, 45:341-354, 1952.

Froehling, D.A., Silverstein, M.D., Mohr, D.N., Beatty, C.W., Offord, K.P., and Ballard, D.J. "Benign Positional Vertigo: Incidence and Prognosis in a Population-Based Study in Olmsted County, Minnesota." *Mayo Clinic Proceedings*, 66(6):596-601, 1991.

Furman, J.M., and Cass, S.P. "Benign Paroxysmal Positional Vertigo." *New England Journal of Medicine*, 341(21):1590-1596, 1999.

Mizukoshi, K., Watanabe, Y., Shojaku, H., Okubo J., and Watanabe I. "Epidemiological Studies on Benign Paroxysmal Positional Vertigo in Japan." *Acta Otolaryngologica, Supplement* (Stockh), 447:67-72, 1988.

Norre, M. "Reliability of Examination Data in the Diagnosis of Benign Paroxysmal Positional Vertigo." *American Journal of Otology*, 16(6):806-810, 1995.

Chapter 2

Structure and Function

To understand the ear, what goes wrong with it, where symptoms come from, and how BPPV tests and treatments work, you should understand something about the ear's normal structure and function. The ear is involved in two important but quite different functions, hearing and balance. Because BPPV affects only balance, this book does not cover hearing.

This chapter consists of basic information. For more in-depth coverage, see "Appendix I: Advanced Balance Concepts."

The Normal Ear

The ear is divided into three parts, the external, middle, and inner ears. (See Figure 2-1.) Only one part, the inner ear, is involved in BPPV.

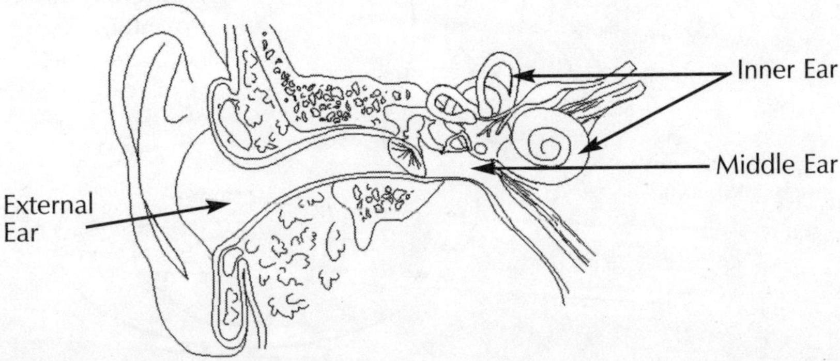

Figure 2-1: The ear. Note the three general parts: the external ear, the middle ear, and the inner ear. (From LifeArt, Corel Gallery Collection, copyright 1994, Williams and Wilkins, a Waverly company, with permission.)

The inner ear itself also has three connected regions—the semicircular canals, the vestibule, and the cochlea—shown in Figure 2-2. (Because the cochlea is involved only in hearing, this book rarely refers to it.)

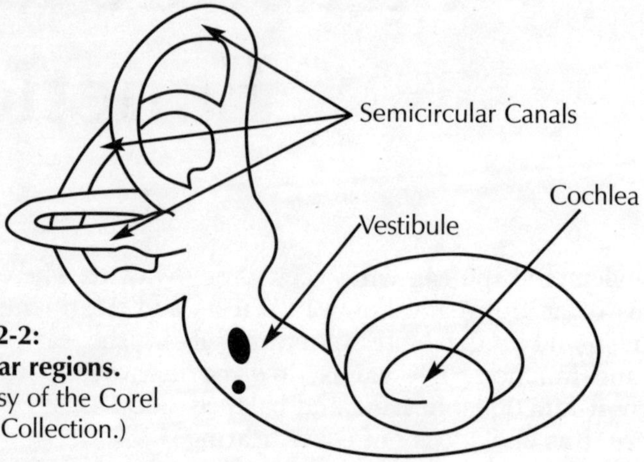

Figure 2-2:
Inner ear regions.
(Courtesy of the Corel Gallery Collection.)

In-depth: The inner ear is also referred to as the labyrinth because of its many interconnected areas and passageways.

Semicircular Canals

You have six semicircular canals, three in each ear.

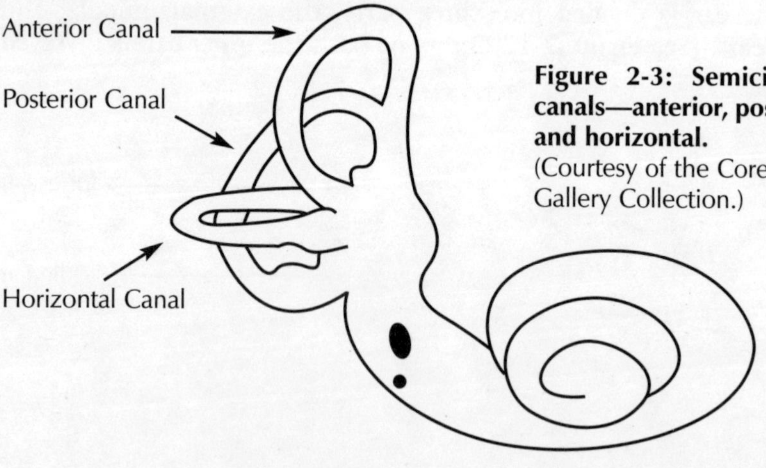

Figure 2-3: Semicircular canals—anterior, posterior and horizontal.
(Courtesy of the Corel Gallery Collection.)

The semicircular canals have several technical names. The anterior canal is also referred to as the superior canal. The horizontal canal is also referred to as the lateral canal, and the posterior canal may also be referred to as the inferior vertical canal. In an upright human, the posterior canals (one in each ear) are the lowest. This lowermost position of the posterior canals is an important factor in BPPV, as explained in the next chapter.

Definitions:
Anterior refers to the front.
Posterior refers to the back.
Lateral refers to either side.
Superior refers to above.
Inferior refers to below.

Near one end, each canal widens to form an ampulla. The short section of canal between the ampulla and the vestibule is called the short arm, while the much longer section is called the long arm. (See Figure 2-4.)

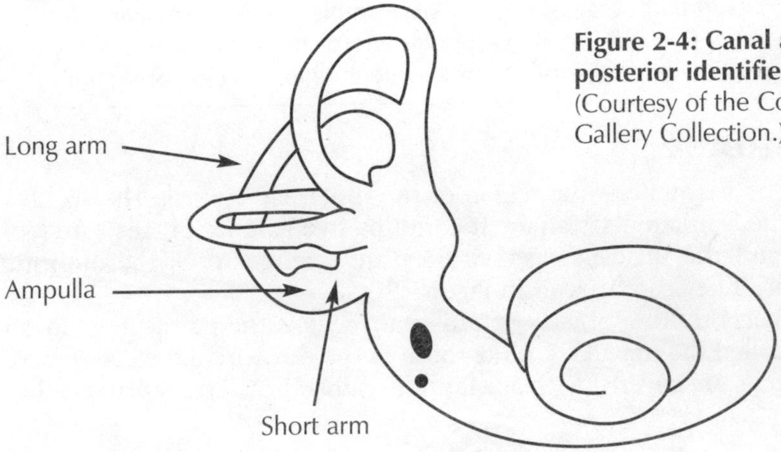

Figure 2-4: Canal arms, posterior identified. (Courtesy of the Corel Gallery Collection.)

Each ampulla houses the cupula of its semicircular canal. The cupula has hair cells on its surface, and these cells send movement information to the brain in the form of nerve impulses.

Definition: A **hair cell** is a specialized epithelial cell that has cilia (hair-like projections) protruding from one end.

In each semicircular canal, the cupula with its hair cells is located near one end of the canal and extends from the floor of the canal to the ceiling, effectively forming a barrier. A fluid called endolymph fills the remainder of each canal. In addition, each canal is surrounded and cushioned by a second fluid, called perilymph.

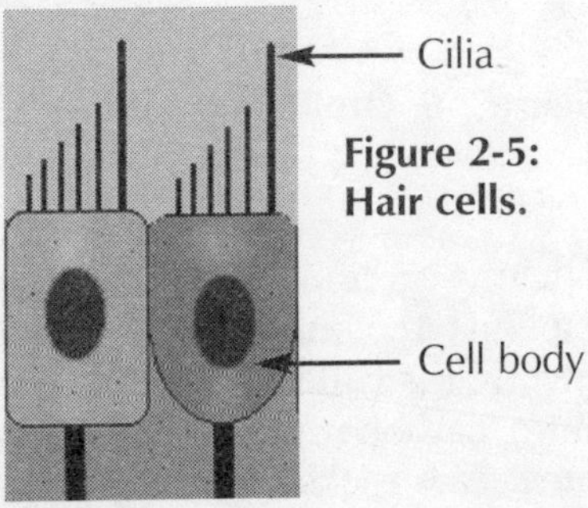

Figure 2-5: Hair cells.

Because of their nearly circular structure, the semicircular canals are responsible for sensing rotational head movement (or rotational body movement that includes the head). The canals move with head turns, but the endolymph in the affected canal creates pressure against the cupula. The resulting distortion of the cupula moves the hair cells, which secrete a neurotransmitter (chemical) that causes a nerve signal to be sent to the brain.

Normally the hair cells of a semicircular canal should only send signals to the brain during rotational head movement, also referred to as angular acceleration. Different head movements (nodding vs. turning vs. tilting) stimulate different canals.

In-depth: Angular acceleration refers to a change in speed along a curved path such as a circle. An example of the sense of angular acceleration is the main vestibular effect you feel on a merry-go-round or spinning around on your feet while dancing or skating.

Vestibule

The vestibule is the region of the inner ear between the cochlea and the semicircular canals. It contains two balance organs, the saccule and the utricle. Together they are referred to as the otolithic organs. They can be seen in Figure 2-6.

Each otolithic organ contains hair cells gathered together in an area called the macula. Unlike those of the semicircular canals, these hair cells are covered with a gelatinous substance. This substance has

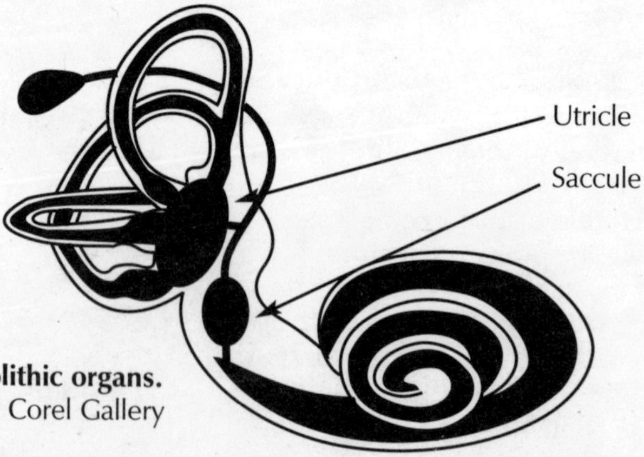

Figure 2-6: Otolithic organs. (Courtesy of the Corel Gallery Collection.)

calcium carbonate crystals embedded in and on it. The next chapter explains the importance of these crystals to BPPV. The gelatinous covering is called the otolithic membrane. (See Figure 2-7.) The calcium carbonate crystals are called otoconia, "otoliths," and sometimes "ear rocks." (See Figure 2-8.)

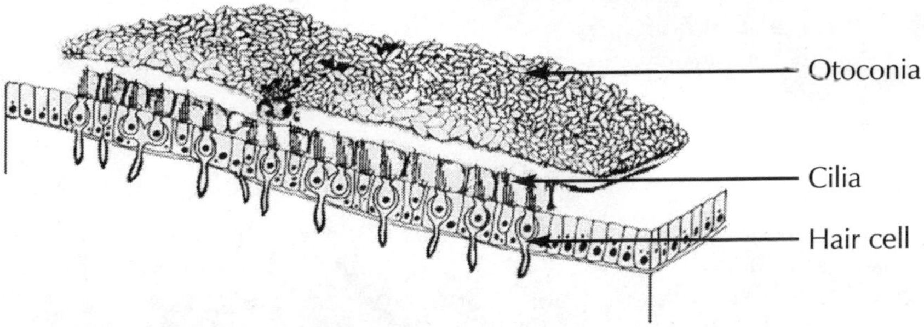

Figure 2-7: Otolithic membrane. (From Lim, D.J. "Formation and Fate of the Otoconia: Scanning and Transmission Electron Microscopy," *Annals of Otolaryngology-Head and Neck Surgery*, 21:23.35, 1973, with permission from Annals Publishing Company.)

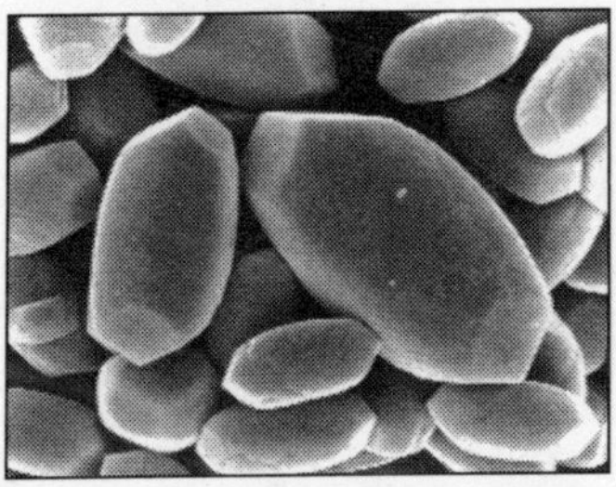

Figure 2-8: Scanning electron micrograph image of otoconia. (From Lim, D.J., "The Development and Structure of the Otoconia," Chapter 10 of *Ultrastructural Atlas of the Inner Ear*, with permission from Butterworth-Heinemann Publishers and Charles G. Wright, Ph.D.)

Normally the otolithic organs sense gravity and linear acceleration. During certain kinds of movement, the combined weight of the otoliths and otolithic membrane bends the hair cells. (See Figure 2-9.)

In-depth: Linear acceleration refers to a change in velocity along a straight line. An example of the sense of linear acceleration is the effect you feel when a jet airplane in which you are riding increases its speed as it zooms down the runway preparing for take-off.

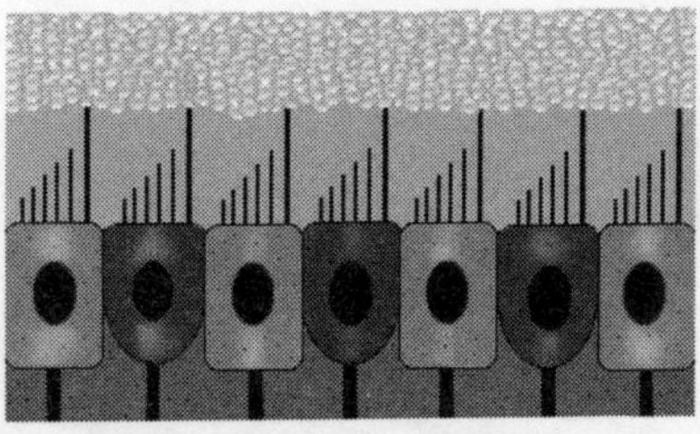

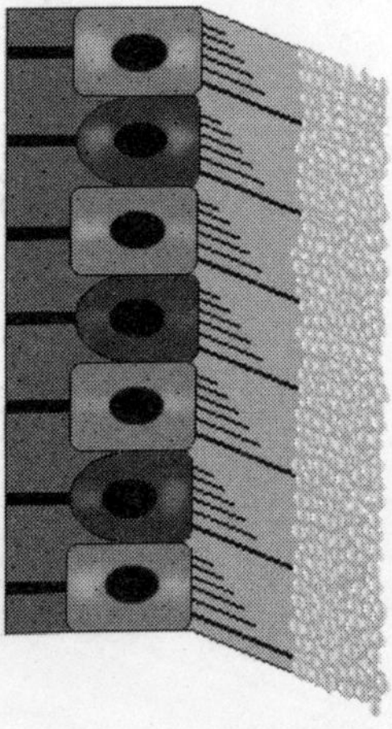

Figure 2-9: Group of hair cells while head is upright and still. Also, group of hair cells, cilia bent by gravity, as head moves to side-lying position.

In-depth: Although each vestibule contains only two of the five balance end organs found in each ear, the word **vestibular** refers to all five.

Vestibulo-Cochlear Nerve

The information collected by the inner ear travels to the brain along the eighth cranial nerve, also called the vestibulo-cochlear nerve, cochleo-vestibular nerve, auditory nerve, or acoustic nerve. In this book, we use the term "vestibulo-cochlear nerve," which states the dual purpose of the nerve. Two branches of this nerve leave the inner ear, the vestibular branch and the cochlear branch; the vestibular branch carries vestibular messages from the five balance end organs, and the cochlear branch carries hearing messages from the organ of Corti.

References

______. *Stedman's Medical Dictionary*. 25th edition. Baltimore: Williams and Wilkins, 1990.

Anson, B.J., and Donaldson, J.A. *Surgical Anatomy of the Temporal Bone*. Philadelphia: W.B. Saunders Company, 1981.

Baloh, R.W. and Honrubia, V. *Clinical Neurophysiology of the Vestibular System*. Philadelphia: F.A. Davis Company, 1990.

Bernat, J.L., and Vincent, F.M. *Neurology: Problems in Primary Care*. Los Angeles: PMIC, 1993.

Berne, R.M., and Levy, M.N. *Physiology*. Third edition. St Louis: Mosby YearBook, 1993.

Cohen, J., and Keshner, E.A. "Current Concepts of the Vestibular System Reviewed: 2.Visual/Vestibular Interaction and Spatial Orientation." *American Journal of Occupational Therapy*, 43:331-337, 1989.

Cummings, C.W., and Harker, L.A. *Otolaryngology-Head and Neck Surgery*. St. Louis: Mosby, 1992.

Guyton, A.C., and Hall, J.E. *Textbook of Medical Physiology*. Philadelphia: W.B. Saunders Company, 1996.

Lim, D.J. "Formation and Fate of Otoconia: Scanning and Transmission Electron Microscopy." *Annals of Otology, Rhinology and Laryngology*, 82:23-35, 1973.

Marieb, E.N. *Human Anatomy and Physiology*. Third edition. Redwood City, Calif.: The Benjamin/Cummings Publishing Company, 1995.

Mira, E. "General View of Vestibular Disorders." *Acta Otolaryngologica, Supplement*, 519:13-16, 1995.

Proctor, B. *Surgical Anatomy of the Ear and Temporal Bone*. New York: Thieme Medical Publishers, Inc., 1989.

Rahn, J.E. *Ears, Hearing, and Balance*. New York: Atheneum, 1984.

Chapter 3

Possible Causes

This chapter discusses three different aspects of BPPV: the event or condition that initially causes the BPPV, the inner ear changes associated with symptoms each time they occur, and the position or movement that causes the individual episodes of vertigo.

Initial Causes of BPPV

A change of some sort must occur to, or in, an individual to set BPPV into motion initially. In about half the people with BPPV, this change is never identified. In the other half, one of several things is thought to be the cause.

Trauma is the leading known cause of BPPV and accounts for about 17 percent of all cases. It is the most frequent cause of BPPV in people under the age of 50. A blow to the head, whiplash, or a blow to the ear have all been known to cause BPPV. Even high-impact aerobics have been reported as an occasional cause.

The second-leading cause of BPPV is change associated with aging; BPPV is much more common in the elderly than in the rest of the population.

BPPV is also frequently seen in people with other inner ear conditions such as vestibular neuronitis, Meniere's disease (11 percent in one study), endolymphatic hydrops, and ototoxicity. It has also been seen after stapedectomy (a type of middle ear surgery) and may occur during or after secondary endolymphatic hydrops from ear infections such as otitis media.

BPPV occurs more frequently in women than in men. The reason for this gender difference is unknown, although at least some experts believe women are more apt than men to seek professional medical care. Another thought, from A. Katsarkas, M.D., is that hormonal differences between men and woman might play a role in the formation of endolymph deposits, especially after menopause.

One rare cause of BPPV is blockage of the anterior vestibular artery, which supplies blood to the utricle of the inner ear.

Inner Ear Changes

Something must occur within the inner ear to bring on a single episode of BPPV symptoms. Over the years, scientists have proposed three theories about what happens in the ear to create the symptoms: (1) otolith dysfunction, (2) cupulolithiasis, and (3) canalithiasis.

Otolith Dysfunction

Up until the 1960s, it was widely believed that BPPV symptoms originated in the utricle, one of the gravity and straight-line movement sensing organs of the inner ear. This theory had a problem, however; it did not account for all the signs and symptoms present in people with BPPV. This theory has mostly disappeared from the medical literature.

Cupulolithiasis

A later theory came about after scientists discovered that at least some people who had been diagnosed with BPPV during their lifetimes had debris attached to the cupula of one or both of their posterior semicircular canals. (See Figure 3-1.)

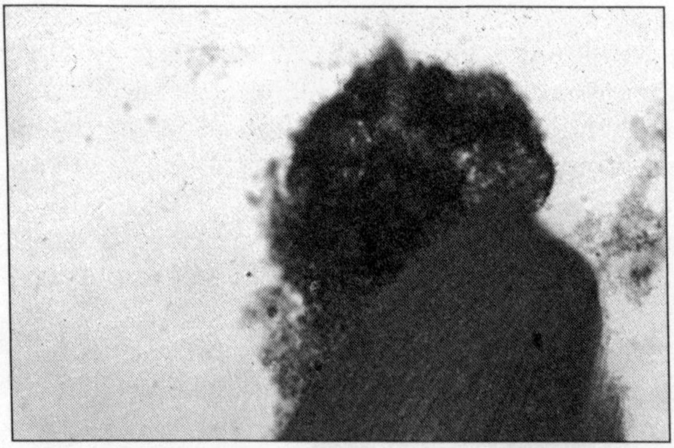

Figure 3-1: Cupular deposits

This condition was named *cupulolithiasis*; "cupulo" refers to the cupula, and "lithiasis" to stones or rock-like substances. The debris was thought to consist of otoconia or "ear rocks" coming from the utricle. Researchers have since found that cupulolithiasis, on occasion, can also occur in the anterior or horizontal canals as well. However, it is most common in the posterior canal, the lowest of the semicircular canals in an upright human. Because the posterior canal is lowest of the three canals during standing or sitting, it's believed that when loose ear rocks are present they will come to rest here because of the effect of gravity.

When debris adheres to a cupula, the hair cells are no longer bent solely by endolymph movement; the weight of the debris can now also bend them. The weighted hair cells respond to changes caused by gravity rather than responding only to changes caused by circular movement. The gravity response causes false information to go to the brain and creates symptoms such as vertigo

---

Note: Most experts think that cupulolithiasis doesn't satisfactorily explain the signs and symptoms of BPPV with changes in head position. If a deposit were clinging to the cupula, they say, its hair cells would send signals to the brain the whole time the head was in an "offending" position, something that does not appear to be the case.

Canalithiasis

A third theory, *canalithiasis*, suggests that debris floating in a semicircular canal causes the symptoms of BPPV. "Canalithiasis" literally means "canal stones," and it is currently the leading theory of BPPV. It's supported by the finding of a white substance floating in the endolymph of the posterior canal in people undergoing surgery for BPPV.

The debris is probably a collection of otoconia, also called canaliths, either loose or grouped together, that have broken away from the utricle. The debris is thought to move when the head moves and to change the pressure on the cupula, bending the hair cells at inappropriate times and sending erroneous signals to the brain.

In-depth: Animal studies show that otoconia can break loose during strong movement, straight and/or curving, such as those that sometimes happen to humans in automobile accidents.

Canalithiasis occurs most frequently within the posterior canal because it is the lowest of the semicircular canals in an upright human, and debris tends to settle. However, canalithiasis can also occur in the anterior or horizontal canals.

Positions That Cause Episodes

H.F. Schuknecht, M.D., in a 1969 article in *Archives of Otolaryngology*, described how the vertigo of BPPV episodes typically begins. "The principle complaint of the patient is the occurrence of sudden attacks of vertigo precipitated by certain head positions," he said. This non-spontaneous feature of BPPV generally sets it apart from other vestibular causes of vertigo. Table 3-1 has examples of changes in head position that might precipitate symptoms in someone with BPPV.

Table 3-1:
Activities That Might Precipitate an Episode of BPPV

Accelerating or decelerating, in a car for example	Nodding your head, as when indicating "yes"
Bending your head to look down	Leaning forward
Bending over	Looking up with the neck extended
Changing a light bulb	Oscillating vertically, for example during jogging or horseback riding
Being moved in a dentist's chair in the pitch plane (the plane in which you nod your head to indicate "yes")	Rapidly turning the head to the side
Drinking, particularly from a can	Rolling over in bed
Getting into bed, lying down	Shaving
Getting out of bed	Straightening up
Getting something from the top shelf	Serving at tennis
Having sexual intercourse	Tilting the head forward
Having your head moved at the hair parlor, particularly having your head tilted into a sink	Tilting the head to the problem side
	Turning or rolling onto the side
	Walking rapidly
	Walking up and down stairs

Here are some descriptions of activities bringing on symptoms:

"The patient reported having episodes of dizziness when lying under a cabinet with his neck extended and looking up, reaching overhead with his neck extended and looking up, looking up and extending his neck while walking down a store aisle, being awakened at night when turning over in bed, and engaging in physical exercise such as jogging."

—C. D. Ford-Smith, P.T., *Physical Therapy*, 1997

"I began to feel that the room was spinning when I woke up in the morning and turned my head from side to side in bed. I also experienced this when I looked up, for example, when reaching for something on a top shelf."

—L.H., letter to the author, 1998

"It also causes what I call the "last inch of pop in the can" problem: namely, I can never finish a can of soda pop because to get the last inch or so would mean I would have to tip my head way back, inducing dizziness."

—S.P., letter to the author, 1998

"Some state that the attack is provoked by a sudden movement of the head to the right or left, or when extending the neck, as in looking upward, and more rarely, when stooping over."

—H.F. Schuknecht, M.D., *Archives of Otolaryngology-Head and Neck Surgery*, 1969

Controversy

Not all MDs working in the field agree on what inner ear changes cause the symptoms of BPPV. Some physicians only accept canalithiasis. Others feel that both cupulolithiasis and canalithiasis exist, cause slightly different sets of positional symptoms, and require different treatments. Recently Honrubia and colleagues have suggested the use of the term "vestibular lithiasis" to refer to both canalithiasis and cupulolithiasis. Rarely an article attributing the symptoms of BPPV to a problem outside the semicircular canal will appear in the medical literature.

References

Baloh, R.W., and Honrubia, V. "Benign Positional Vertigo: Clinical and Oculogyric Features in 240 Cases." *Neurology*, 37:371-378, 1987.

Baloh, R.W., Jacobson, K., and Honrubia, V. "Horizontal Semicircular Canal Variant of Benign Positional Vertigo." *Neurology*, 43:2542-2549, 1993.

Brandt, T. "Positional and Positioning Vertigo and Nystagmus." *Journal of Neurological Sciences*, 95:3-28, 1990.

Brandt, T., and Daroff, R.B. "Physical Therapy for Benign Paroxysmal Positional Vertigo." *Archives of Otolaryngology*, 106:484-485, 1980.

Cawthorne, T. "Positional Nystagmus." *Annals of Otology*, 63:481-490, 1954.

Dix, M.R., and Hallpike, C.S. "The Pathology, Symptomatology and Diagnosis of Certain Common Disorders of the Vestibular System." *Proceedings of the Royal Society of Medicine*, 45:341-354, 1952.

Dornhoffer, J.L., and Colvin, G.B. "Benign Paroxysmal Positional Vertigo and Canalith Repositioning: Clinical Correlations." *American Journal of Otology*, 21:230-233, 2000.

Epley, J.M. "The Canalith Repositioning Procedure: For Treatment of BPPV." *Otolaryngology-Head and Neck Surgery*, 107(3):399-404, 1992.

Epley, J.M. "Positional Vertigo Related to Semicircular Canalithiasis." *Otolaryngology-Head and Neck Surgery*, 112:154-161, 1995.

Fife, T.D. "Recognition and Management of Horizontal Canal Benign Positional Vertigo." *American Journal of Otology*, 19:345-351, 1998.

Ford-Smith, C.D. "The Individualized Treatment of a Patient with Benign Paroxysmal Positional Vertigo." *Physical Therapy*, 77(8):848-855, 1997.

Gacek, R.R. "Cupulolithiasis." *Advances in OtoRhinoLaryngology*, 28:80-85, 1982.

Gyo, K. "Benign Paroxysmal Positional Vertigo as a Complication of Postoperative Bedrest." *Laryngoscope*, 98:332-333, 1988.

Hall, S.F., Ruby, R.R., and McClure, J.A. "The Mechanics of Benign Paroxysmal Vertigo." *Journal of Otolaryngology*, 8(2):151-158, 1979.

Harada, Y., and Sufimoto, Y. "Metabolic Disorder of Otoconia After Streptomycin Intoxication." *Acta Otolaryngologica*, 84:65-71, 1977.

Honrubia, V., Baloh, R.W., Harris, M.R., and Jacobson, K.M. "Paroxysmal Positional Vertigo Syndrome." *American Journal of Otology*, 20:465-470, 1999.

Katsarkas, A. "Paroxysmal Positional Vertigo: An Overview and the Deposits Repositioning Maneuver." *American Journal of Otology*, 16(6):725-730, 1995.

Katsarkas, A. "Benign Paroxysmal Positional Vertigo: Idiopathic Versus Post-Traumatic." *Acta Otolaryngologica*, 119:745-749, 1999.

Lanska, D.J., and Remler, B. "Benign Paroxysmal Positioning Vertigo: Classic Descriptions, Origins of the Provocative Positioning Technique and Conceptual Development." *Neurology*, 48:1167-1177, 1997.

Lindsay, J.R., and Hemenway, W.G. "Postural Vertigo Due to Unilateral Sudden Partial Loss of Vestibular Function." *Annals of Otolaryngology-Head and Neck Surgery*, 65:692-706, 1956 .

Moriarity, B., Rutka, J., and Hawke, M. "The Incidence and Distribution of Cupular Deposits in the Labyrinth." *Laryngoscope*, 102:56-59, 1992.

Schuknecht, H.F. "Cupulolithiasis." *Archives of Otolaryngology-Head and Neck Surgery*, 90:113-126, 1969.

Parnes, L.S., and McClure, J.A. "Free-Floating Endolymph Particles: A New Operative Finding During Posterior Semicircular Canal Occlusion." *Laryngoscope*, 102(9): 988-992, 1992.

Schuknecht, H.F. "Cupulolithiasis." *Archives of Otolaryngology-Head and Neck Surgery*, 90:113-126, 1969.

Thomas, C.L. *Taber's Cyclopedic Medical Dictionary*, 15th edition. Philadelphia: F.A. Davis Company, 1985.

Welling, D.B., Parnes, L.S., O'Brien, B., Bakaletz, L.O., Brackmann, D.E., and Hinojosa, R. "Particulate Matter in the Posterior Semicircular Canal." *Laryngoscope*, 107(1):90-4, 1997.

Chapter 4
Types of BPPV

The majority of BPPV cases are of the "textbook" variety. The episodes are unaccompanied by other inner ear problems. They affect only the posterior canal in one ear. The debris is floating within the canal. The symptoms occur in a limited number of positions. This BPPV is "self-limiting" (goes away by itself in a few weeks to months) or responds quickly to treatment. If your BPPV has just begun, chances are you will have this simplest form and will not have to think about patterns, intensity, canals other than the posterior, or debris.

However, for a small number of people BPPV does not follow the usual pattern. Canals other than the posterior can be involved, and BPPV can affect multiple canals simultaneously in more than one ear. Several patterns and intensity levels are possible, and the BPPV can be accompanied by other inner ear problems that cause significant complications.

Physicians sometimes classify BPPV by pattern, intensity, the canal(s) affected, and the involvement of one ear or both ears. Some also categorize it by debris.

Canals

BPPV can affect any of the three semicircular canals in either ear and can affect more than one canal simultaneously. It can also exist in both ears at the same time. The posterior canal is by far the most common site of trouble; the anterior canal is next, and the horizontal is last.

Researchers report varied numbers for the horizontal canal type ranging from 1 percent to 22 percent of all people with BPPV; however, the range between 1 and 4 percent is the most commonly quoted. Anterior canal BPPV accounts for around 4 percent. The rest occur in the posterior canal.

When BPPV occurs in a canal other than the posterior, it is referred to as a variant. The horizontal type, for example, would be referred to as the horizontal variant of BPPV.

Ears

Not only can the BPPV affect canals other than the posterior, it can also occur in only one ear or in both. When affecting one ear only, it is referred to as unilateral. If affecting both ears simultaneously, it is referred to as bilateral.

Pattern

H.F. Schuknecht, M.D., categorized BPPV cases by the symptom patterns he observed in his patients: *self-limiting, remitting/recurring,* or *persistent*. The self-limiting type stops spontaneously (without treatment) within a few weeks or, possibly, months. The remitting/recurring type involves symptoms that come and go over weeks to years. The third type, persistent BPPV, does not go away without surgical intervention.

> "I've learned to sleep on three pillows. I haven't lain on my right side in two years."
>
> —B.C., letter to the author, 1998

Intensity

BPPV can also be classified by symptom intensity. According to J.M. Epley, M.D., someone with occasional episodes of positional vertigo and no symptoms between episodes has *mild BPPV*. A case of *moderate BPPV* includes an episode of vertigo every time a particular position is assumed and might involve constant lightheadedness. *Extreme BPPV* involves vertigo produced by most head movements and in which nausea is constant.

> ". . . for the following 23 months I lived in a constant state of mild disequilibrium. Every time I turned in bed to the right, I experienced violent vertigo. . . . My vision lacked its usual sharpness. I frequently found myself walking around unaware that I was wearing my reading glasses since it made little difference one way or the other. . . . I was exhausted all the time."
>
> —Mary B., R.N., *More Stories and Strategies*, 1995

Debris

Some physicians believe that both canalithiasis and cupulolithiasis can occur. Canalithiasis refers to otoconia free-floating in a canal, while cupulolithiasis refers to otoconia adhering to a cupula. Recently it has been suggested that the term *vestibular lithiasis* be used to refer to both canalithiasis and cupulolithiasis.

Controversy

A significant number of physicians do not agree about the existence of the different patterns and intensities of BPPV, particularly the persistent and extreme varieties suggested by Schuknecht and Epley. Many believe if the symptoms are constant or nearly so, the disorder must be something other than BPPV. This book takes no position on the issue and will present information from medical journals about both the less severe and more severe varieties.

Complications from Other Inner Ear Disorders

Unfortunately, BPPV can occur with, or be caused by, other vestibular problems such as vestibular neuronitis, ototoxicity, perilymph fistula, Meniere's disease, endolymphatic hydrops, and inner ear syphilis. BPPV accompanied by another vestibular problem will usually have many symptoms beyond those of unaccompanied BPPV. Both positional vertigo and the symptoms of the other disorder will be present at various times in varying degrees. BPPV accompanied by another inner ear disorder can cause a great deal of suffering and create significant problems in both diagnosis and treatment.

Important Points

Most cases of BPPV are self-limiting, mild, unilateral, and involve only the posterior canal. They are not difficult to diagnose or treat. More complicated cases occur, however, but are not as common.

References

______. *More Stories and Strategies*. Portland, Ore.: Vestibular Disorders Association, 1995.

Epley, J.M. "BPPV: Diagnosis and Management," *Vestibular Update*, 8:1-4, 1992.

Fife, T.D. "Recognition and Management of Horizontal Canal Benign Positional Vertigo." *American Journal of Otology*, 19:345-351, 1998.

Herdman, S.J. *Vestibular Rehabilitation* Philadelphia: F.A. Davis, Company, 2000.

Honrubia, V., et al. "Paroxysmal Positional Vertigo Syndrome." *American Journal of Otology*, 20:465-470, 1999.

Schuknecht, H.F. "Cupulolithiasis." *Archives of Otolaryngology-Head and Neck Surgery*. 90:113-126, 1969.

Wolf, J.S., et al. "Success of the Modified Epley Maneuver in Treating Benign Paroxysmal Positional Vertigo." *Laryngoscope*, 109:900-903, 1999.

Chapter 5

Signs and Symptoms

To know BPPV, you must understand the nature, strength, frequency, duration, and impact of its symptoms. Not all people experience BPPV in the same way; symptoms depend on the type of BPPV. People with the mild, self-limiting type may experience attacks of vertigo with no other symptoms or lingering effects. Symptoms for other people might linger for a short while after an episode of vertigo. On rare occasion, someone with extreme and/or persistent BPPV might have more constant symptoms, not just bursts of vertigo. Symptoms such as sleepiness during the day, memory problems, and malaise can also occur as indirect consequences of this disorder.

Attack

In the quote below, Dix and Hallpike describe a "textbook" case of posterior canal BPPV:

> "The story given by the patient is characteristically that the giddiness comes on when he lies down in bed and when he turns over in bed, or when such a position is taken up during the day; for instance, in lying down beneath a car or in throwing the head backward to paint a ceiling. The patient sometimes, although not always, recognizes that the onset of the vertigo is associated with the critical position and will say that he does his best to avoid it."
>
> —Drs. M.R. Dix and C.S. Hallpike, *Annals of Otology*, 1952

A typical attack begins a few seconds after someone with BPPV assumes the offending position, and it usually lasts from 5 to 10 seconds. It can last longer than this but never more than 60 seconds. Although an attack of BPPV is of short duration, it can still have several signs and symptoms including vertigo, nystagmus, nausea, and fear.

Vertigo

Definition: Vertigo is the perception of movement (either of yourself or of objects around you) that is not occurring, or is occurring differently from what you perceive.

The name of this disorder includes the word "vertigo" for good reason. Vertigo is the most profound symptom and the one most likely to cause a person to seek medical attention. People who experience this vertigo often describe it as strong, sometimes violent.

> "The sensation of vertigo is always of short duration, usually about 5 to 10 seconds, which helps to distinguish this condition from other vestibular disorders. Because of the intensity of the vertiginous sensation, the patients commonly assign a longer duration to the attack, and careful questioning may be required to elicit a reliable history . . .."
>
> —H.F. Schuknecht, M.D., *Archives of Otolaryngology*, 1969

The type of vertigo most commonly associated with BPPV is spinning. Spinning vertigo can also be referred to as whirling, circling, rotating, rotational, rotatory, or turning.

> "I began to feel that the room was spinning when I woke up in the morning and turned my head from side to side in bed."
>
> —L.H., letter to the author, 1998

> "Whenever I would bend down to look to the side or look up and over my shoulder, I would experience the feeling of violent horizontal spinning. The entire sensation would last approximately 20 seconds."
>
> —T.M., letter to the author, 1998

Others types of vertigo, though, can also occur, including rocking, dropping, tumbling, falling, tilting, and movement in a straight line.

> "I will begin to have a slow, forward tumbling, just like I'm somersaulting down a hill in slow motion."
>
> —S.P., letter to the author, 1998

Vertigo occurs because your brain expects consistent vestibular signals from all five vestibular organs in each ear. A sudden, inconsistent signal from one canal creates a mismatch between information from one ear and information from the other. The false signal will also not match information going to your brain from your eyes and from sensors in your muscles and joints. This information mismatch confuses the brain and creates the sensation of vertigo.

Nystagmus

Nystagmus is present with the vertigo, and it starts and stops in unison with it. Nystagmus is an abnormal jerking of the eyes. In posterior canal BPPV this jerking is a twisting or rotary movement. You may feel eye movement, and your vision may appear to be bouncing or twisting during the few seconds that nystagmus is present. Someone examining your eyes can see the nystagmus when you experience an episode of vertigo.

As odd as it might sound, the inner ears and the eyes have a close relationship. They are physically connected via the vestibulo-ocular reflex (VOR), and when one ear undergoes a change, nystagmus can occur. See more in "Appendix A: Advanced Balance Concepts."

Nausea

Some people experience nausea during their short bouts of vertigo. Vomiting can occur but is rare since an episode of vertigo is short.

Note: Prolonged vomiting is highly unusual with BPPV. If you have vomiting that persists longer than two hours, call your doctor to report it.

Fear

Fear and all that accompanies it can also occur during an episode of BPPV. You might experience cold sweat, anxiety, trembling, increased heart rate, palpitations, and a dry mouth. The autonomic nervous system is responsible for this "fight or flight" response to danger and stress and, at times, vertigo. This system will "rev up" your body to stand and fight or to run as fast as possible out of harm's way. You will experience an increased heart rate and rate and depth of breathing, pupil dilation, goose bumps, sweating, release of adrenaline, decrease in urine production, decrease in saliva, increased blood flow to certain areas and decreases to others, and a general increase in the metabolic rate (the speed at which the body operates).

This "rev up" is an excellent response if a dog attacks you, for example. It allows you to "hit the ground running." But, if you are not physically threatened, changes in the autonomic nervous system can be disturbing and even bad for your general health. They make an episode of vertigo feel extremely serious and body-wide rather something limited to the inner ear.

Typical BPPV Experience

The following account is typical of those given by people with a diagnosis of BPPV:

"Whenever I would bend down and look to the side or look up and over my shoulder, I would experience the feeling of violent horizontal spinning. I could also feel my eyes moving rapidly from side to side. The entire sensation would last approximately 20 seconds. The sensation was very similar to the spinning and nystagmus cause by the injection of water into my ears during an ENG.

"The spinning vertigo was also entirely predictable based on my head movements, and I was able to protect myself because I knew that certain movements were likely to induce it, such as bending down in the shower to get shampoo. Accordingly, I would take precautions to prevent falling, and I would make a point of turning around to talk to people rather than looking over my shoulder."

—T.M., letter to the author, 1998

After an Attack

Most people with BPPV can resume their previous activities immediately after an episode of positional vertigo. They might feel a need to avoid the position that brought on the signs and symptoms, and they might feel lingering fear or anxiety. On rare occasion, they might feel unsteady for a while after an episode.

Between Attacks

If you have a self-limiting and/or mild form of BPPV, you will not experience vertigo, nystagmus, nausea, imbalance or other vestibular symptoms between attacks. You should be able to function at the same levels you did before the BPPV.

Some people with BPPV will on occasion experience fear, anxiety, worry, have questions about their capabilities. Much of this is normal and should not noticeably alter their ability to function. On rare occasion, these problems may cause people to become depressed.

If your BPPV occurs frequently in bed, you may experience further problems including sleepiness during the day, malaise, decreased alertness, poor memory, decreased motor abilities, confusion, and suspicion.

Sometimes people will sleep sitting up or will fix pillows in their beds to prevent moving into positions that produce vertigo. These efforts may interfere with sleep and may produce sleepiness during the day and other symptoms linked to sleep disturbance.

Secondary problems created by BPPV can also disturb sleep. Fear, anxiety, and/or anger can make falling asleep difficult, and depression can cause you to awaken from sleep prematurely.

Controversy

Not all doctors believe BPPV has more persistent or severe forms, and they will make a diagnosis other than BPPV if the symptoms go beyond those discussed above. You can find further information about these symptoms in "Appendix II: Possible Symptoms of Severe/Persistent BPPV."

The Impact of BPPV Symptoms

Many people with the self-limiting form of BPPV aren't affected greatly by their symptoms. Some are troubled greatly for only a short time (days to weeks). Unfortunately, persistent BPPV can turn the lives of some people literally upside down with profound and prolonged symptoms. In these cases, the disorder disturbs most facets of life.

> "These episodes of dizziness resulted in poor job performance and occasional nights of interrupted sleep."
>
> —C. D. Ford-Smith, P.T., *Physical Therapy*, 1997

> "The simplest things like trying to buy groceries, doing laundry, cleaning the bathrooms, my husband has to do now. I do have good times and actually get to leave the house for short times."
>
> —S.S., letter to the author, 1998

> "I am afraid to sleep on the side that always caused me to have vertigo. I hesitate to dance fast and twirl, bend over with my head lower than my knees as I pull weeds, look in file drawers, etc."
>
> —Cheryl K., *More Stories and Strategies*, 1995

> "My sense of confidence and freedom of movement are memories I long for."
>
> —V.H., letter to the author, 1998

> "Unless you have experienced it, you have no idea how hard just living is."
>
> —V.N., letter to the author, 1998

"I think back, and all the frustration and confusion and terror come back to me."

—Y.S., letter to the author, 1998

"I had to brace myself to take a shower, and many nights I would just skip brushing my teeth to avoid the head position and movement."

—Y.H., letter to the author, 1998

"Some patients complained of severe curtailment of sexual activities. This was particularly marked in women who could not lie supine without developing vertigo."

—J.M. Epley, M.D., *Otolaryngology-Head and Neck Surgery*, 1980

Few activities in life require no head movement. In someone with vertigo initiated by every head movement, no activity is free of symptoms. BPPV can make someone feel too sick, fearful, and/or spatially confused to perform the simplest tasks.

Horizontal Canal Variant

Horizontal canal BPPV occurs much less often than posterior canal BPPV, and far, far less has been written about it. It was not described in the medical literature until 1985.

Like posterior canal BPPV, horizontal canal BPPV is characterized by vertigo lasting less than 60 seconds and is brought on by a change in head position. The vertigo of horizontal canal BPPV is said to be more intense than the posterior canal variety.

Other symptoms associated with but not limited to horizontal canal BPPV include the illusion of walking on pillows, nausea (sometimes constant and sometimes in response to head movement), and unsteadiness.

Most commonly, rolling onto either side or from side to side while in bed precipitates the vertigo. The vertigo can occur any time you move your head in the direction sensed by the horizontal canal; for example, when you shake your head "no."

As with the posterior canal variant, the impact varies greatly from person to person and depends on the strength and frequency of the vertigo and other symptoms.

References

______. *More Stories and Strategies*. Portland, Ore.: Vestibular Disorders Association, 1995.

Baloh, R.W., Honrubia, V., and Jacobson, K. "Benign Positional Vertigo: Clinical and Oculographic Features in 240 Cases." *Neurology*, 37(3):371-378,1987.

Cohen, H.S., and Jerabek, J. "Efficacy of Treatments for Posterior Canal Benign Paroxysmal Positional Vertigo." *Laryngoscope*, 109:584-590, 1999.

Dix, M., and Hallpike, C. "The Pathology, Symptomatology and Diagnosis of Certain Common Disorders of the Vestibular System." *Annals of Otology*, 61:987-1016, 1952.

Epley, J.M. "New Dimensions of Benign Paroxysmal Positional Vertigo." *Otolaryngology-Head and Neck Surgery*, 88:599-605, 1980.

Fife, T.D. "Recognition and Management of Horizontal Canal Benign Positional Vertigo." *American Journal of Otology*, 19(3):345-351, 1998.

Ford-Smith, C.D. "The Individualized Treatment of a Patient with Benign Paroxysmal Positional Vertigo." *Physical Therapy*, 77(8):848-855, 1997.

Herdman, S.J. "Advances in the Treatment of Vestibular Disorders." *Physical Therapy*, 77(6):601-618.

Levinson, H. N. *Phobia Free: A Medical Breakthrough Linking 90 Percent of all Phobias and Panic Attacks to a Hidden Physical Problem*. New York: M. Evans and Company, 1986.

Nuti, D., Vannucchi, P., and Pagnini, P. "Benign Paroxysmal Positional Vertigo of the Horizontal Canal: A Form of Canalithiasis with Variable Clinical Features." *Journal of Vestibular Research*, 6(3):173-184, 1996.

Potter, P.A., and Perry, A.G. *Basic Nursing: Theory and Practice*. St. Louis: Mosby. 1995.

Schuknecht, H.F. "Cupulolithiasis." *Archives of Otolaryngology-Head and Neck Surgery*, 90:113-126, 1969.

Chapter 6

Diagnosing BPPV

If you have BPPV and no other inner ear problems, diagnosing it is straightforward in the broad majority of cases. Your physician takes your history, examines you, tests you for BPPV, and makes a diagnosis. This chapter covers the history, examination, and BPPV testing for all variants of BPPV. In a small number of cases, more testing is required or ordered. You can find explanations of these further tests in Appendix C, "More About Tests."

History

Your physician needs to hear your story in order to form an idea of what is wrong and which tests to request. Also, she or he must know your history in order to interpret test results accurately; vestibular disorders cannot always be distinguished from one another solely on the basis of testing. Without complete knowledge of the symptoms and the rest of your story, the test results may not lead to an accurate diagnosis. Your medical history includes all the information about your past or present that can help your doctor understand your current health status and assess the problem for which you seek treatment. This means information about the following:

- Your general health
- Ear infections or ear problems you had in the past
- Any diseases, problems, accidents, or injuries you have had
- What drugs you are taking or have taken in the not too distant past
- Any treatments you may be undergoing and the purpose for the treatments
- Any special diet you are on and why
- Your symptoms
- What you feel during an episode of vertigo
- What you were doing when the symptoms first appeared
- When the symptoms occur
- If the symptoms are spontaneous or if some specific activity or circumstance brings them on
- How long the symptoms stay

- How strong they are
- How often they come
- How many times you have had them
- If they include nausea or vomiting
- If anything makes the symptoms better
- If anything makes them worse
- If you have ever had anything like them
- If you have any relatives with similar symptoms
- The general health of your closest relatives

Examination

Generally your doctor will first want to know whether your symptoms result from a problem that can cause great harm in the immediate future; thus the examination will cover a lot of areas. Luckily, most causes of dizziness, including BPPV, will not directly cause loss of limb or life. In fact, all inner ear causes of vertigo are considered "benign." In this context, benign means they won't kill you even though they may disrupt your life.

An otolaryngologist's examination of someone with dizziness usually focuses on the following:

- Ear
- Hearing (not affected by BPPV but can be affected by other vestibular disorders)
- Nose/sinuses and throat
- Brain and nervous system
- Eye movement
- Balance and movement

In-depth: Testing and conscious manipulation

Sometimes people undergoing examination and testing feel their symptoms and the problems created by them have been minimized or ignored by the health care professionals they have encountered. In an attempt to make their symptoms and difficulties visible during testing or examination, they may choose not to walk or stand in place to the best of their ability, or they may allow themselves to fall when they could prevent it.

Exaggeration of disability can lead to the wrong diagnosis and treatment, or it can cause doubt in the examiner's mind about whether not you have a physical problem. It's in your best interest during an examination or testing procedure to carry on to the best of your ability. Don't yield to the temptation to "show them how you feel."

Hearing

An audiologist may check your hearing before you see the doctor, or your otolaryngologist might have you listen to a tuning fork(s) placed behind your ears or on your forehead. You might be asked to compare sounds or say when a sound disappears. Hearing loss is not part of BPPV, but some other inner ear disorders can affect hearing. Testing helps rule those other possibilities in or out. (Appendix C contains more about hearing tests.)

Ear

The external ear canal can be examined directly for obstruction by things such as wax, infection, or foreign bodies. The tympanic membrane (ear drum) can be checked for holes (perforations), signs of fluid or infection in the middle ear, and for a middle ear growth called a cholesteatoma.

Nose, Sinuses, and Throat

The nose, sinuses, and throat are checked for inflammation, swelling, infection, or any other abnormality.

Brain and Nervous System

Your doctor will check the function and condition of your brain indirectly by checking a number of things such as how well you can answer questions, how your eyes move, what your eye pupils look like and how they react to light, and how you move muscles around your face. The doctor may also check your muscle strength and coordination and your reflexes and might also test your senses of smell, taste, touch, and vision.

Balance and Movement

For a quick look at your balance function, your doctor will have you stand with your feet side by side and eyes closed or with one foot in front of the other and might also have you "march in place," stand on one foot, or stand on your toes. The doctor may also push you a bit while you are standing. He or she will have you walk in your normal way, may ask you to walk by placing one foot in front of the other or heel to toe, and may have you walk backwards. Possibly, you may be asked to stand on a cushion or walk on something soft.

Eye Movement

Your doctor will observe your eyes for nystagmus while your head is still, when you are moving your head, when you are following his finger with your eyes, and possibly when he or she is moving your head or when you are in different positions. The examiner may also perform a Dix-Hallpike test. See below for a full description of this test. He or she may check your vision with a standard wall chart while you stand still or possibly while you move your head. You might be asked to put on a pair of glasses or goggles. These magnify your eyes for the examiner and force you to look through lenses you cannot focus with. This prevents you from fixing your vision on something, which would make it difficult for the doctor to see eye movement abnormalities that might be present.

Feeling Dizzy: Understanding and Treating Vertigo, Dizziness and Other Balance Disorders by Brian W. Blakeley, M.D., and Mary-Ellen Siegel, M.S.W. (MacMillan, 1995), includes an excellent in-depth description of the kind of examination a newly dizzy person might undergo.

Your doctor will use both the information you provide and the results from your examination to either determine a diagnosis or select further testing such as the Dix-Hallpike test to help in the determination. More information about tests can be found in Appendix C.

BPPV Testing

Two tests exist for diagnosing BPPV, the Dix-Hallpike for the posterior and anterior types, and the roll test for the horizontal variant.

Special Instructions

To be useful, these tests must be done in a specific manner. You must follow the tester's directions and allow him or her to position you freely. You will need to maintain certain testing positions even if they cause vertigo. In fact, the occurrence of vertigo during a test will help your doctor decide why you sometimes experience vertigo at other times. Because the vertigo and nystagmus of BPPV tend to decrease as the day goes on, try to schedule your tests early in the day.

After the Tests

This testing can cause nausea, fatigue, and a temporary off-balance sensation. Plan to have someone drive you home from the testing, or allow enough time to recover before driving.

Dix-Hallpike Maneuver

Introduced in 1952 by the two British physicians for whom it is named, the Dix-Hallpike maneuver has been widely used ever since. Your doctor might perform the maneuver as part of your initial examination, or it might be done by itself or as one of a series of tests performed by a technician, audiologist, or other tester.

What It Is Like

The Dix-Hallpike maneuver is a positioning test during which you are moved rapidly into specific positions and your eyes are observed for nystagmus. You must keep your eyes open during this test.

Here is the original description (*Proceedings of the Royal Society of Medicine*, Vol. 45, p. 349) of the positioning test by Dix and Hallpike:

"The patient is first seated upon the couch (exam table) with the head turned to one side and the gaze fixed upon the examiner's forehead. The examiner then grasps the patient's head firmly between his hands and briskly pushes the patient back into the critical position (the head lowered 30 degrees below the level of the couch and turned some 30 to 45 degrees to one side)."

Generally the test is done first with the head turned 30 to 45 degrees to one side, followed by the head turned 30 to 45 degrees to the opposite side, finally with the head in the center. This series of position changes may be repeated once or twice. Each position change, from sitting to lying, takes less than two seconds. If the changes were done more slowly, the vertigo and nystagmus might not

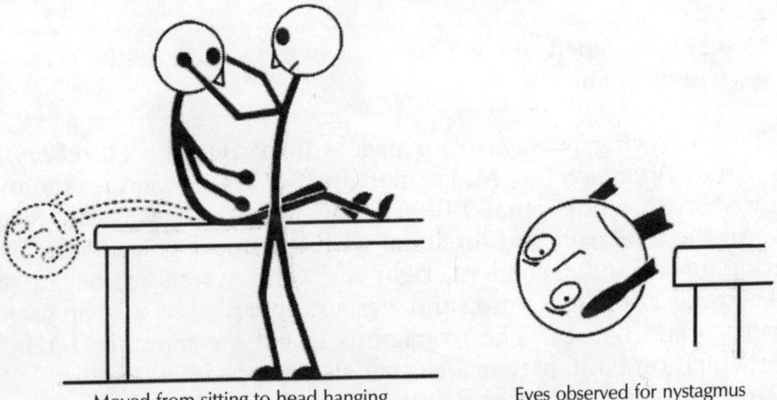

Figure 6-1: Dix-Hallpike maneuver. (From Carmichael, E.A., Dix, M.R., and Hallpike, C.S. "Pathology, Symptomatology and Diagnosis of the Organic Affections of the Eighth Nerve System," *British Medical Bulletin*, 12:146-152, 1956, with permission.)

occur, and the test finding would be negative even if BPPV were present.

Proper observation of eye movement is important to this test. Methods of observing or recording nystagmus vary greatly from one testing center to the next. Here are some possibilities:

- You wear no special equipment. An observer watches your eyes.
- You wear special glasses (Frenzel lenses) that don't allow you to focus on your surroundings and that improve the tester's view of your eyes.
- You wear special goggles that can't be seen through. They contain infrared cameras that record eye movement.

Positive Test Signs

A positive test for BPPV consists of several findings, as follows:

- Rotary and/or twisting nystagmus and vertigo occur 2 to 15 seconds after you assume the head-hanging position.
- A decrease in the nystagmus and vertigo occurs after 2 to 30 seconds in the position.
- The nystagmus and vertigo have a crescendo-decrescendo pattern. (They increase then decrease in intensity.)
- Vertigo and nystagmus are gone within 60 seconds, usually less.
- Usually a reverse in the direction of the nystagmus and a slight feeling of vertigo occur after you sit back up.
- The nystagmus fatigues (decreases gradually in severity) with repeated testing.

Note: Many experts think a diagnosis of BPPV requires the presence of nystagmus.

The following passage from page 136 of *Balance Disorders: A Case Study Approach* by J.M. Furman and S.P. Cass describes the nystagmus of posterior canal BPPV: "The nystagmus was upbeating (toward the forehead) and torsional with the upper poles of the eyes beating toward the dependent (right ear). The nystagmus began several seconds after positioning and was accompanied by a strong sense of vertigo and nausea. The nystagmus lasted for about 15 seconds, after which time the patient's vertigo also stopped."

In right-sided posterior BPPV, the vertigo and nystagmus occur with the head lowered and turned to the right. They occur in left-sided BPPV with the head lowered and turned to the left.

The opposite occurs in the anterior canal variant of BPPV. Vertigo and nystagmus occur with the head lowered and turned to the right in the left-sided anterior canal variant, for example.

What the Test Shows

Both posterior canal BPPV and the anterior canal variant of BPPV can be diagnosed through the use of the Dix-Hallpike maneuver. If the test is done and interpreted properly, a negative test means that the nystagmus of BPPV was not present at the time of the test. This does not mean BPPV has never been present, only that it was not active during the test.

Horizontal Canal Test

What It Is Like

The horizontal canal test used by some testers involves a positioning maneuver during which you lie flat on the examining table and the tester either turns your head or your entire body quickly to the right. You remain in this position for about 30 seconds, then the tester returns your head or body to the original starting position (lying flat). You maintain this second position for a short time, then the tester turns your head or body quickly to the left, pauses for a while, and returns your head or body to the starting position (lying flat).

Proper observation of eye movement is one key to this test. Methods of observing or recording eye movements used by different testers can vary greatly. Here are some possibilities:

- You wear no special equipment. An observer watches your eyes.
- You wear special glasses (Frenzel lenses) that don't allow you to focus on your surroundings and that improve the tester's view of your eyes.
- You wear special goggles that can't be seen through. They contain infrared cameras that record eye movement.
- You wear sticky-patch electrodes connected to a device that records your eye movements electronically.

Positive Test Signs

Perhaps because this test is much newer than the Dix-Hallpike maneuver, experts disagree about what constitutes a positive test. Some authorities have suggested the following:

- Horizontal nystagmus and vertigo occur in one to five seconds on the affected side.
- The nystagmus changes direction, and a lesser vertigo occurs when the head is placed in the opposite position.
- The nystagmus and vertigo usually last less than two minutes on the affected side.

What the Test Shows

This test can only show if the horizontal variant of BPPV is present. If the test is done and interpreted properly, a negative test shows that the horizontal canal variant of BPPV was absent during the test. This does not mean it has never been present.

General Preparation for These Tests

Follow the instructions of your doctor or the testing center about medications. Go to the test fully rested, and wear something comfortable. Women will be more comfortable if not wearing a dress or skirt.

If you have a neck or back problem, inform your doctor and the staff at the testing place before going for testing. If you have a false eye, need glasses to see beyond the tip of your nose, use contact lenses, or have a visual problem called strabismus, tell the tester before the start of the test.

The staff of the doctor's office or the testing center should provide you with complete instructions about preparation, when to show up, and how much time to allow for testing. In general, anti-vertigo drugs and any other drugs that could affect the test results are stopped 24 to 48 hours before these tests. Drugs such as meclizine (Antivert and Dramamine Less Drowsy formula), dimenhydrinate (Dramamine Original formula), Phenergan, Compazine, and painkillers can interfere with the test. If you have any questions about drugs, call your doctor's office or the testing center staff for clarification.

Testing and Drugs

It is important to follow your doctor's instructions about what drugs can be taken or not taken before and during testing and for how long. When health professionals refer to medications or drugs in this context, they mean over-the-counter drugs like aspirin or street drugs such as cocaine as well as drugs prescribed by a doctor.

Your doctor will not want you to take medications that can interfere with testing. He or she also will not want you to stop taking any medications, such as insulin, heart drugs, or blood pressure medications essential for treating other conditions. If you have conditions that require medication, discuss them with your doctor.

Some drugs can cover up abnormalities that must be observed or measured during testing, and other drugs can create abnormalities. Table 6-1 lists some common drugs known to interfere with accurate testing.

Table 6-1: Drugs That May Impede Testing

Alcohol	Lithium
Amitriptyline	Marijuana
Antivert (meclizine)	Methadone
Aspirin	Nicotine gum
Ativan (lorazepam)	Quinine
Barbiturates	Sedatives in general
Benadryl	Tegretol (carbamazepine)
Dilantin (phenytoin)	Tobacco
Elavil	Tranquilizers in general
Imipramine	Valium (diazepam)
Librium (chlordiazepoxide)	Xanax (alprazolam)

Allergy

Some vestibular tests use sticky patches, electrodes that are stuck to the body, usually on the face and or head. These usually contain water, glycerol, and polyacrylic acid (containing sodium sulfonate groups). If you're allergic to any of these, notify your doctor's office and the testing center.

Important Points

The diagnosis of BPPV is straightforward in most people seeking care from an experienced and knowledgeable neurotologist, an inner ear balance expert. There are tests for all three types of BPPV: posterior, anterior and horizontal. Sometimes your doctor will request other tests beyond those described in this chapter. More information about these tests can be found in Appendix C.

References

Baloh, R.W., Honrubia, V., and Jacobson, K. "Benign Positional Vertigo: Clinical and Oculogyric Features in 240 Cases." *Neurology*, 37:371-378, 1987.

Baloh, R.W., Yue, Q., Jacobson, K.M., and Honrubia, V. " Persistent Direction-Changing Positional Nystagmus: Another Variant of Benign Positional Nystagmus?" *Neurology*, 45:1297-1301, 1995.

Dix, M.R., and Hallpike, C.S. "The Pathology, Symptomatology and Diagnosis of Certain Common Disorders of the Vestibular System." *Proceedings of the Royal Society of Medicine*, 45:341-354, 1952.

Fife, T.D. "Recognition and Management of Horizontal Canal Benign Positional Vertigo." *American Journal of Otology*, 19:345-351, 1998.

Furman, J.M., and Cass, S.P. *Balance Disorders: A Case-Study Approach*. Philadelphia: F.A. Davis, Company, 1996.

Lanska, D.J., and Remler, B. "BPPV: Classic Descriptions, Origins of the Provocative Positioning Technique, and Conceptual Developments." *Neurology*, 48:1167-1177, 1997.

Mohr, D.N. "The Syndrome of Paroxysmal Positional Vertigo: A Review." *Western Journal of Medicine*, 145:645-650, 1986.

Nuti, D., Vannucchi, P., and Pagnini, P. "Benign Paroxysmal Positional Vertigo of the Horizontal Canal: A Form of Canalolithiasis with Variable Clinical Features." *Journal of Vestibular Research*, 6(3):173-184, 1996.

Schuknecht, H.F. "Cupulolithiasis." *Archives of Otolaryngology-Head and Neck Surgery*, 90:113-126, 1969.

Chapter 7

Treatment—Introduction

Several treatment approaches are in use for BPPV ranging from doing nothing to performing surgery. BPPV differs from most other vestibular disorders in that effective medical (non-surgical) treatments are available that can stop symptoms without risk to hearing and/or balance in the majority of people. Some medical treatments have, on occasion, been able to stop the episodes of vertigo in people with long-standing BPPV in as little as one treatment session.

A common approach in the past was to do nothing since BPPV disappeared spontaneously in many people. No studies prove that a delay in treatment will affect the eventual outcome, but some experts in the field think that the longer the BPPV goes untreated the more difficult it is to treat successfully. As a consequence, some experts treat BPPV immediately to relieve suffering instead of using the wait-and-see approach.

Doctors in the U.S. use a number of treatments. No standard treatment exists, although one (with a number of variations), the canalith repositioning procedure, is used most widely. Table 7-1 lists treatments.

Table 7-1: Treatment Methods

Debris Removal
Canalith repositioning procedure
Brandt-Daroff exercises
Semont maneuver
Horizontal canal variant maneuvers

Relief from Additional Symptoms
Vestibular Rehabilitation

Surgery
Canal plugging
Singular neurectomy

Temporary Suppression of Symptoms with Drugs*
Anti-anxiety/anti-vertigo drugs
Anti-nauseant drugs
Anti-motion-sickness drugs
Miscellaneous drugs

*Drugs are seldom used to treat BPPV. For descriptions of specific drugs, see Appendix D.

About Surgery

Many textbooks and other sources of information about vestibular disorders focus heavily on surgical treatments because surgery is technically demanding and needs lots of explaining, not because it is common. Doctors sometimes suggest surgery for BPPV when all medical treatments have failed, when hope of spontaneous resolution has dimmed, and when a patient is so severely affected that he or she cannot function in a reasonably normal way in everyday life. Surgery for BPPV should never be the first treatment option offered.

Few people with BPPV, perhaps 1 percent, will ever require surgery for symptom control. Chapter 10 has information for people forced to consider a surgical option.

Treatment Choice

The treatment your doctor suggests to you may depend on many things, including the following (not listed in order of importance):

- your doctor's philosophy about whether or not to treat the apparent cause of BPPV or the symptoms or both
- your doctor's opinion of the cause
- your doctor's experience with observing and treating patients like you
- what your doctor learned in medical school and during residency training about BPPV
- which semicircular canal or canals are affected
- whether another inner ear problem accompanies the BPPV
- your age and physical condition
- the condition of your neck and back
- the degree of your disability
- whether one or both ears are affected
- the severity of the vertigo
- the type and severity of symptoms between attacks
- your job/your home activities and responsibilities
- the demands upon your physician
- your financial or insurance situation
- the length of time you've had BPPV

Difficulties Finding Effective Treatment

Finding an effective treatment is difficult at times because:

- Not all doctors are familiar with medical treatments for BPPV.
- Some health care professionals offering medical treatments have limited experience and training in their use.

- The event that causes BPPV to begin in the first place is unknown. This makes finding a permanent solution difficult in some cases.
- Treatments for BPPV have, for the most part, not been subjected to controlled human studies.

Removing vs. Relocating Debris

You might wonder why doctors don't simply enter the sick semicircular canal and remove the debris thought to be causing BPPV. Getting rid of the debris is easier said than done. Entering the ear surgically to remove debris or to inject a chemical to dissolve the debris would probably result in hearing loss or deafness and could also damage the vestibular parts of the ear.

The most commonly used BPPV treatments attempt to relocate debris to non-sensitive places within the inner ear and to do this without risk to hearing or balance.

Disclaimer

VEDA and the author do not mean to endorse or disavow the many treatments mentioned in this book. The treatments mentioned here have already been discussed in scientific and popular journals, magazines, newsletters, and other publications. We have included them so that you can learn about their large number and great diversity. Some of these treatments have been widely used in the United States, where this book was written and published; others have not. What treatment, if any, you choose should depend upon consultations with your physician.

Chapter 8

Debris Movement

The illustrations and explanations in this chapter are meant to help you understand the nature and purpose of specific BPPV treatments. During some of these treatments, a health care professional must observe and correctly interpret eye movement to assure correct timing of movements and to prevent injury. Attempting these treatments on your own could cause increased symptoms or, worse, serious injury to your back, neck and/or head from poor alignment or a fall. In certain situations, it could also damage your inner ear. *Consult with a physician trained in the diagnosis and treatment of BPPV to determine if any of these treatments might be of value in your particular case. Don't do them on your own unless instructed to by a physician.*

Canalith Repositioning Procedure (CRP)

The canalithiasis theory of BPPV states that free-floating debris can migrate into a semicircular canal and cause short episodes of vertigo when it moves within the canal. This theory is the rationale behind the CRP treatment. Since the debris is free-floating, it's thought that this procedure can help move the debris from the sensitive area (semicircular canal) into a place where it won't cause vertigo.

CRP can be used to treat BPPV of the posterior semicircular canal or the anterior semicircular canal. Most people undergoing the procedure do so for posterior canal BPPV; therefore most graphics and explanations focus on this canal.

A piece of debris in a semicircular canal is also referred to as a canalith, which literally means a canal rock (rock = lith). The debris is thought to consist of calcium carbonate crystals that have detached from the utricle in the vestibule of the inner ear.

The CRP is also sometimes referred to as:

- the Epley maneuver or maneuvers
- the repositioning maneuver for BPPV
- deposits repositioning
- the deposits repositioning maneuver

- the canalith repositioning maneuver
- canalith releasing
- the particle repositioning maneuver
- canalith redistribution

John M. Epley, M.D., first described the canalith repositioning procedure in a medical journal in 1992. The original procedure and many variations are currently in use and are referred to, at times, as the Epley maneuver or maneuvers. Because many of these procedures differ significantly from the maneuver suggested by Epley, this book will use the term "canalith repositioning procedure."

How It Works

Through a series of head position changes, the CRP moves the canaliths from the canal to the utricle. Once in the utricle, the canaliths may re-adhere to the otolithic membrane, dissolve, be broken up perhaps by vestibular dark cells, or move some place where they can't cause symptoms.

Figure 8-1: Posterior canal and utricle. (From LifeArt, Corel Gallery Collection, copyright 1994, Williams and Wilkins, a Waverly company, with permission.)

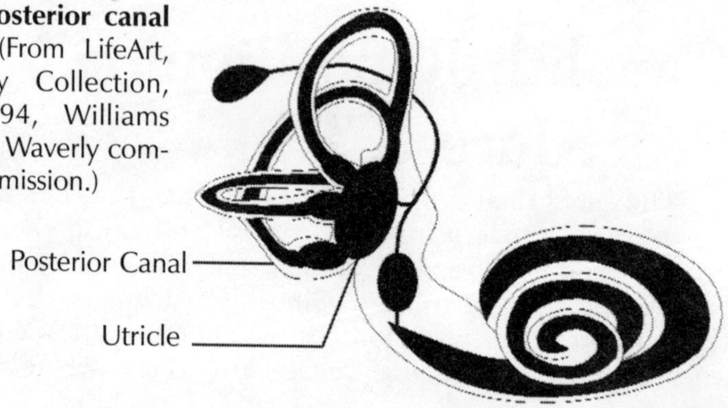

The Procedure

If you have the CRP, usually a health care professional (medical doctor, physical therapist, audiologist, occupational therapist, or possibly someone else) will move your head through a series of positions. The exact method varies considerably from one professional to another.

The descriptions and drawings below are from medical journals and books, and they show that the CRP is performed at various clinics in a great variety of ways. Much disagreement exists among physicians and others about the best way to do the treatment with the greatest chance of success.

The procedure, as originally described by Epley in 1992 (Figure 8-2), consisted of the following:

- pre-medication with diazepam or Transderm-Scop given with its peak effect timed to help block nausea during the procedure
- a series of head position changes in which eye movements were closely watched
- use of a vibrator during head-position changes to help break up and move the debris
- instructions to the patient to keep his or her head upright for 48 hours after the procedure to keep the debris from re-entering the posterior canal

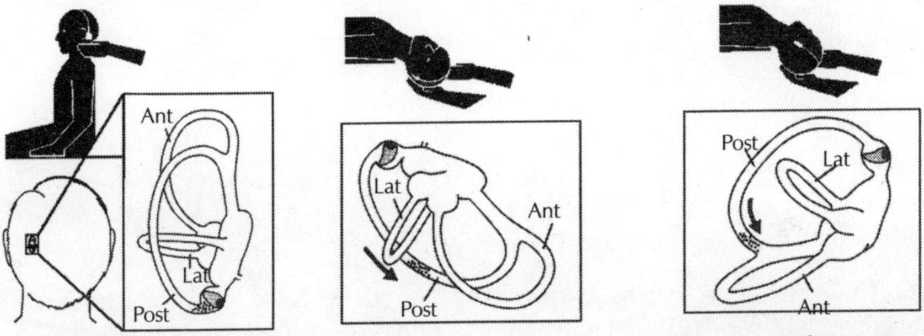

1. Starting position. Debris can be seen to the left of the posterior semicircular canal cupula. The white headband is the vibrator.
2. The first position change begins to move the debris away from the cupula.
3. The second position change moves the debris further away from the cupula.

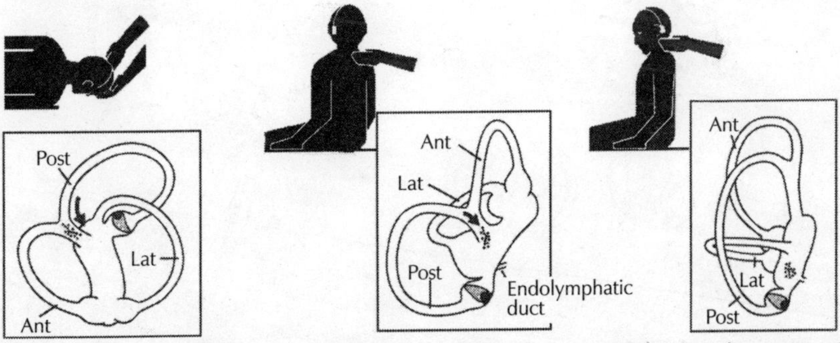

4. The third position change moves debris almost out of the posterior semicircular canal.
5. The debris passes out of an area called the common crus and begins to enter t h e utricle in the vestibule.
6. The debris has moved completely out of the canal and into the utricle.

Figure 8-2: Treatment of the left ear. From Epley, J.M. "Canalith Repositioning Procedure," *Otolaryngology-Head and Neck Surgery,* 107(3):401, 1992. (Courtesy of the publisher.)

The CRP, as described by Welling in 1998 (Figure 8-3), consisted of a series of head position changes in which eye movement was watched. The procedure sometimes included gentle shaking of the head during the position changes, and it required the patient to keep his or her head elevated at least 45 degrees above horizontal for 48 hours afterwards.

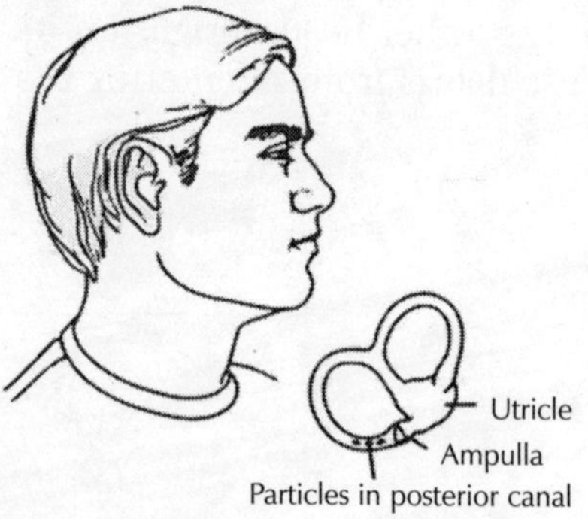

1. The procedure begins with your head upright for 10 minutes to allow the debris to accumulate in the posterior semicircular canal, the lowest area.

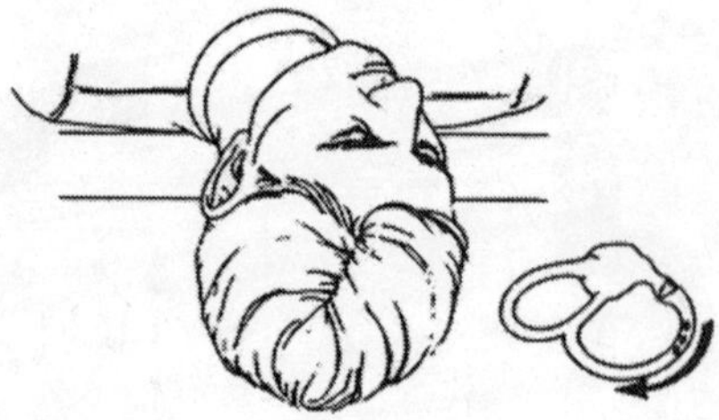

2. You lie back with your head supported over the edge of the table.

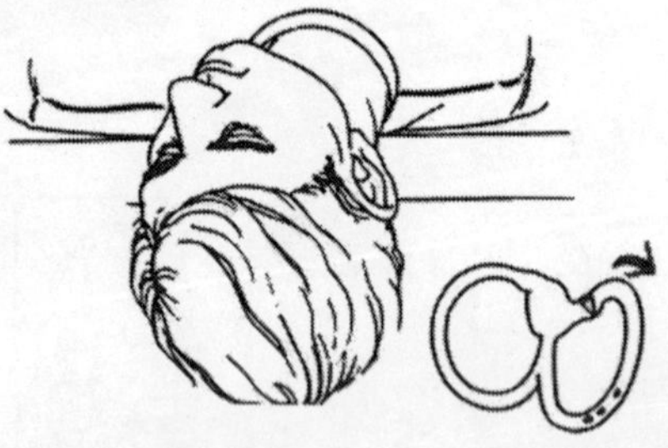

3. Your head is rotated to the opposite side to move the debris further away from the cupula of the sick canal.

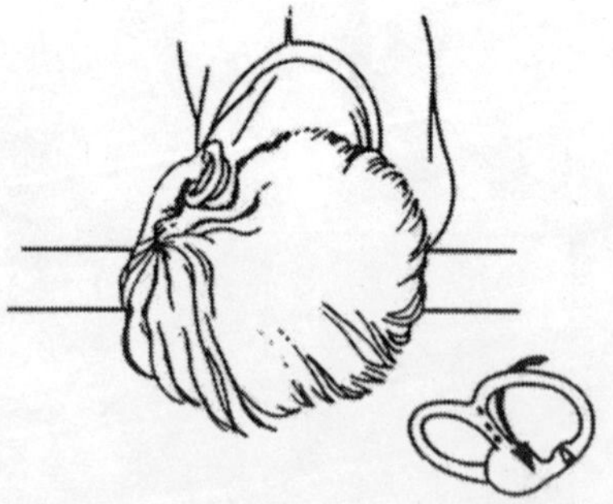

4. Your head and body are positioned to move the debris through the common crus into the utricle.

Figure 8-3: Treatment of the right posterior semicircular canal. From Welling, D.B., and Burnes, D.C., "The Incidence and Distribution of Cupular Deposits in the Labyrinth." *Laryngoscope*, 104:947, 1994. (Courtesy of Lippincott, William, and Wilkins.)

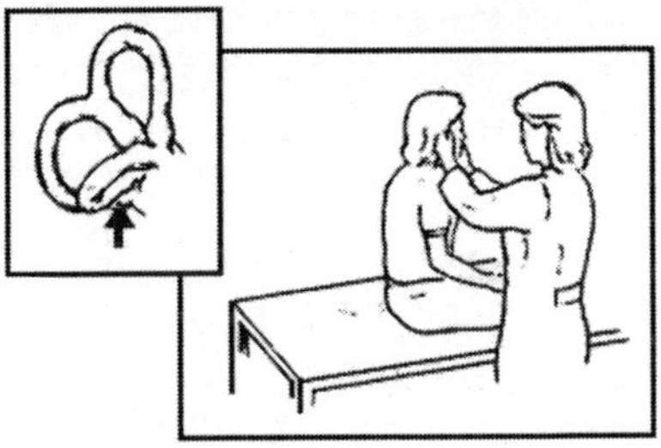

1. Starting position.

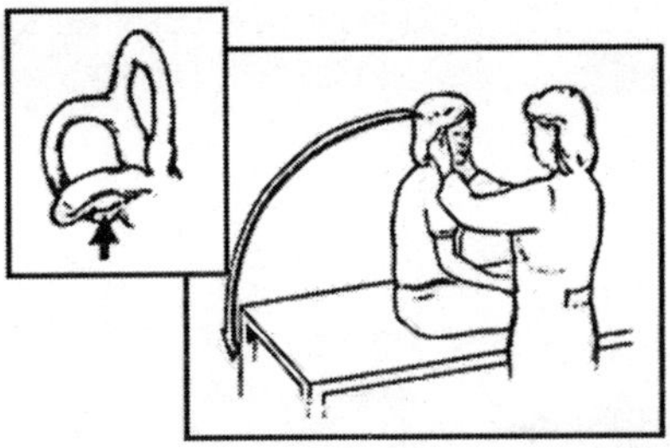

2. Your head is turned, and then you are moved into a lying position.

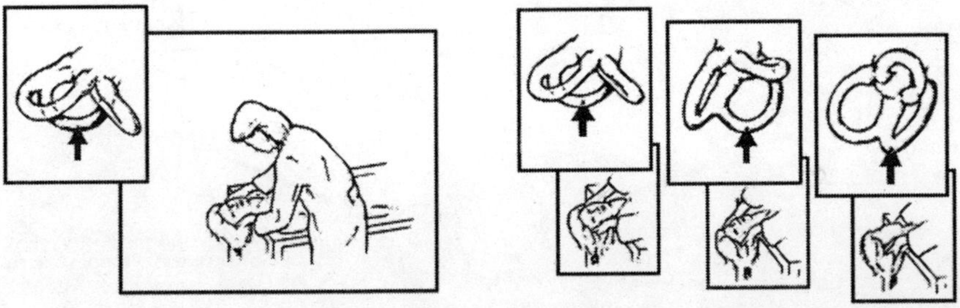

3. You lie back with your head supported over the edge of the table. The debris begins to move away from the cupula. Your head is moved from right ear down to left ear down. The debris moves further from the cupula.

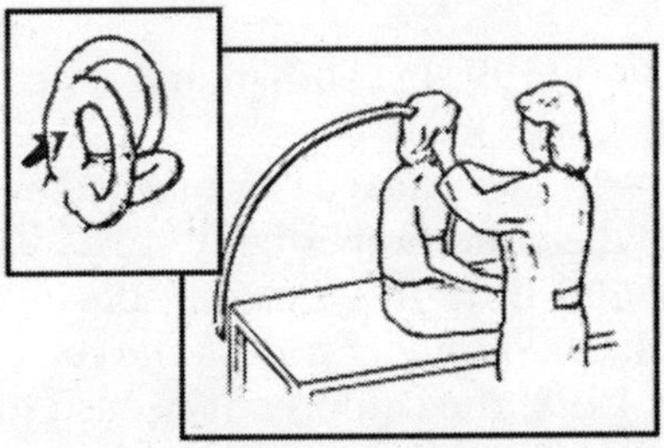

4. You are returned to a sitting position. The debris has moved into the utricle.

Figure 8-4: Another treatment of the right posterior semicircular canal. From Herdman, S., et al., "Single Treatment Approaches to BPPV, *Archives of Otolaryngology-Head and Neck Surgery*, 119:452, 1993. (Courtesy of the publisher.)

As described by Herdman in 1997 (Figure 8-4), the CRP consisted of a series of timed changes in head position. The patient was instructed to keep his or her head elevated and to wear a cervical collar for 48 hours after the procedure to avoid neck bending of any type.

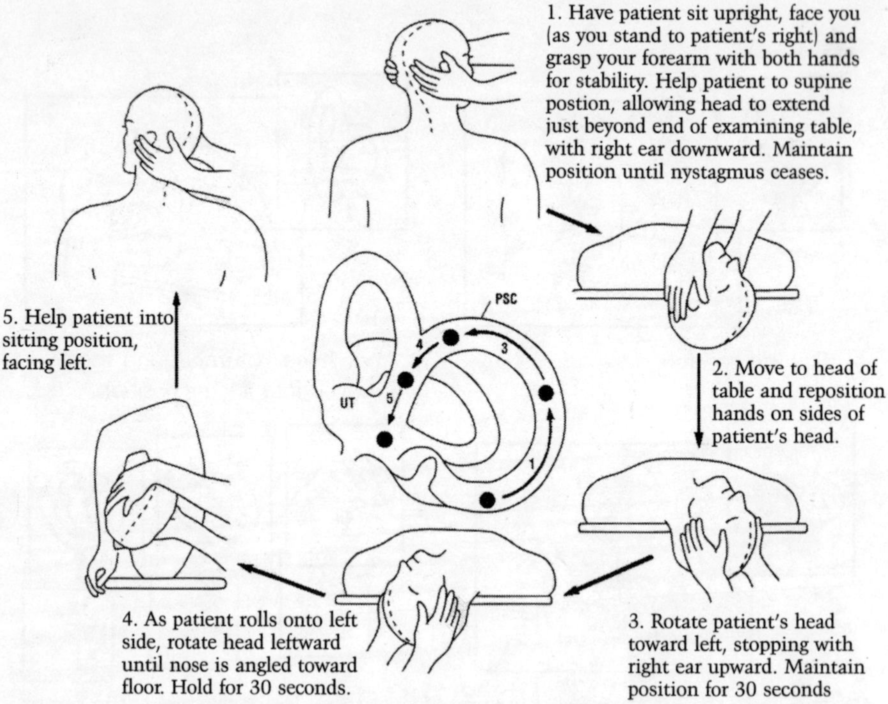

Figure 8-5: Treatment of the posterior semicircular canal. *Conn's Current Therapy*, 47th edition, Philadelphia: W.B. Saunders Co., p. 839, 1995. (Courtesy of the publisher.)

The procedure of Baloh (1995) is shown and described in Figure 8-5.

Furman and Cass in 1998 also described a "head over heels" CRP, which can be done when the proper equipment is available. Instead of moving the body and head in ways that create unusual demands on the neck and back, the provider moves the patient's entire body in a seated position. In 1998, the equipment needed to do this was available in the U.S. in only two places.

Personal Accounts

"I have had BPPV since I was 7 years old, when I was knocked off a see-saw. I am now 55 years old, and am happy to report that this year I found relief from the sudden spinning as a result of subtle changes in head position that has plagued me all of my life.

"Using the utmost patience with my panicky feelings, Daniel (the audiologist) maneuvered my head in various positions while using a vibrator to redistribute the canaliths. The actual procedure took just half an hour. It was a particular relief when he assured me that as soon as I became dizzy from the head positions, he could and did relieve the dizziness. After a second follow-up visit I haven't been back to see him in six months."

—J.S., "Epley Maneuver for BPPV," *On the Level*, Fall 1998

"In October 1997, it happened again. I awoke to a spinning bedroom. Terrified, I called and got right in to the doctor and with one treatment I walked out of his office with no vertigo. The vertigo never came back."

—J., "Epley Maneuver," *On the Level*, Winter 1998

Success Rates

Most studies have found that for posterior canal BPPV the CRP, in its many variations, succeeds in the broad majority of people. These studies are difficult to combine for an exact success statistic because the procedures differ greatly, as do the measurements and definitions of success. In general the reported success rates range between 85 and 95 percent after one or more tries.

Few studies report on the outcome of CRP for the anterior variant of BPPV. Those that do so mention success rates as low as 50 percent.

"I had the 'Epley Maneuver' done three times. I felt noticeably better after the first time but really didn't get rid of the 'marbles rolling around' feeling until after the third time."

—V.N., letter to the author, 1999

Preventing Immediate Recurrence

Most doctors and others carrying out the CRP tell patients to avoid certain head positions for 24 to 48 hours. During this time, the debris presumably moves some place where it can't create symptoms and most likely reattaches to the otolithic membrane, dissolves, or is broken down by vestibular dark cells.

Not for Everyone

If you have a perilymph fistula, detached retina (a structure inside the eye), hydrocephalus or any other condition increasing the pressure in and around your brain, cervical arthrosis, vertebrovascular insufficiency, chronic neck or back problems or esophageal reflux, you may be excluded from having the CRP. Your doctor may also advise against the CRP if you have had a recent head, neck, or back injury. If you experience neck pain during the procedure, your provider may stop doing the CRP to avoid injuring your neck.

Possible Problems

The CRP might cause the following problems:

- Debris moved by the CRP might lodge in another canal such as the horizontal, thus causing the horizontal variant of BPPV.
- In theory, the CRP movements might injure the neck or back, particularly in people with pre-existing neck and back problems.

Why It Might Not Work

CRP might not work for any of the following reasons:

- The diagnosis of BPPV was incorrect.
- The wrong canal was treated.
- The procedure was performed incorrectly.
- Other inner ear problems are also causing symptoms; therefore improvement in BPPV symptoms goes unnoticed.
- Vibration is needed to make the procedure work.
- The debris is adhering to the cupula rather than floating in the canal.
- Floating debris is not the problem.
- More debris floats into the posterior semicircular canal after the procedure.
- The angles between the canal and the other parts of the inner ear are not normal, and this prevents appropriate movement of the debris.

If It Doesn't Work

If the treatment fails to cure the problem, it can be repeated as many times as needed. The option of trying a different treatment is also still available. One physician put it this way:

> "It may be worthwhile to consider a different maneuver with patients who are not responding to treatment after two attempts with an initial maneuver. An appropriate protocol for patients who fail treatment with the Epley maneuver is to first try the maneuver with mastoid oscillation. If this fails, another maneuver, such as Semont's maneuver should be attempted."
>
> —Wolf, et al., *Laryngoscope*, 1999

Brandt-Daroff Exercises

In 1980, Drs. T. Brandt and R.B. Daroff suggested a set of exercises for BPPV to be done every three hours throughout the day and extending until two days after the bouts of positional vertigo had ended. In their words, they treated people by "challenging them with the precipitating head positions on a repeated and serial basis."

How They Work

According to Brandt and Daroff:

> "The presumed mechanism for this therapy is the loosening and ultimate dispersion of degenerated otolithic particles from the cupula of the posterior semicircular canal."
>
> —*Archives of Otolaryngology*, 1980

This treatment is based upon the cupulolithiasis theory of BPPV. It is hoped that repetitive movement will loosen debris from the cupula and prevent further episodes of positional vertigo.

Others in the field have suggested these exercises also might work through habituation.

Definition: Habituation is the repetitive presentation of a stimulus to the brain to reduce the brain's response to it. The stimulus, in this case, is the nerve signal arriving in the brain from a sick ear. If the stimulus is frequent, the brain may reduce its response, and the vertigo, nausea, and other BPPV symptoms may lessen or stop.

How They Are Done

The procedure as described by Brandt and Daroff is as follows:

1. Sit on the edge of a bed, with eyes closed, halfway between the foot and head of the bed.
2. Move into a side-lying position with the head positioned as shown in the figure below, and stay there until the vertigo ends.
3. Return to sitting position; stay there for 30 seconds.
4. Move onto the opposite side with the head positioned as shown in the figure below, and stay there for another 30 seconds. (If vertigo occurs on this side as well, stay in the position until it stops.)
5. Return to the sitting position.
6. This sequence of position changes is repeated until the position change does not bring on vertigo.
7. Steps one through six are repeated 5 times two or three times a day
8. The exercises are repeated until vertigo is not experienced at all for two days.

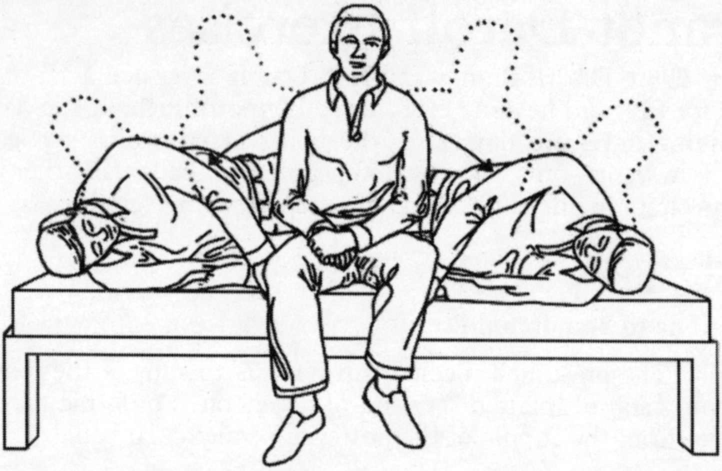

Figure 8-6: Brandt-Daroff exercises. Adapted from Brandt, T., and Daroff, R.B., "Physical Therapy for Benign Paroxysmal Positional Vertigo," *Archives of Otolaryngology-Head and Neck Surgery,* 106(8):484-485, 1980.

Some people express concern about falling from the bed during these exercises. To eliminate this possibility, you can do the exercises on the floor.

Success Rates

The 1980 account of Brandt and Daroff described the effect of the exercises on 67 people.

Complete relief occurred in 66. In two people, the BPPV later returned but again disappeared after the exercises. The one person not experiencing relief was later diagnosed with a different inner ear problem, a perilymph fistula.

Another Use

Some experts prescribe these exercises for use in the weeks and months after performing CRP in the hopes that it will prevent a BPPV relapse.

Semont Maneuver

How It Works

The force of a series of head/body movements detaches debris from the cupula and moves it out of the semicircular canal, or it moves free-floating debris particles out of the semicircular canal into the utricle. Once the debris is out of the semicircular canal, the episodes of vertigo stop.

The Procedure

If you are treated with the Semont maneuver, a health-care professional, medical doctor, physical therapist, audiologist, occupational therapist, or someone else with appropriate training will move you through a series of position changes, beginning with the sitting position. From there you will be moved rapidly onto the side opposite your side with the BPPV, and your head will be rotated so your nose touches the bed. Then you will be moved back to a sitting position and then onto your opposite side, and your head will be rotated so your face is upward. Then you will be moved from that side to the opposite side in one smooth movement, and your head will be rotated so your face is pointed down. During these maneuvers, the health-care professional will observe your eyes for telltale movements. You will maintain the last position for 10 minutes, and then you will be moved once more into the position that previously caused vertigo to determine if your vertigo has vanished.

Preventing Immediate Recurrence

To prevent immediate recurrence, the health professional will instruct you to keep your head vertical for a time, often 48 hours. In 1999, Semont recommended one week and suggested avoiding activities such as tennis and golf for a further two weeks.

Not for Everyone

The same limitations might apply to the Semont procedure as to the CRP (page 61-62.)

Possible Problems

Possible problems include an episode of vertigo during the procedure. Also, in theory the neck or back might be injured, particularly in people with pre-existing neck and back problems.

Why It Might Not Work

The Semont maneuver might not work for any of the following reasons:

- The diagnosis of BPPV was incorrect.
- The wrong canal was treated.

- The procedure was performed incorrectly.
- Other inner ear problems are also causing symptoms; therefore improvement in BPPV symptoms go unnoticed.
- More debris floats into the posterior semicircular canal after the procedure.
- Floating debris is not the reason for the vertigo.
- Debris is the problem, but the maneuver fails to remove it.
- The angles between the canal and the other parts of the inner ear are not typical, and this prevents the desired debris movement.

Horizontal Canal Treatments

Five medical treatment approaches have been described in the medical literature since 1993 for the horizontal canal variant of BPPV. This variant was first described in 1985 and, according to published statistics from separate studies, accounts for about 1 percent, about 5 percent, or about 22 percent of all cases of BPPV. Information about treatments—their success rates, possible complications, numbers needed, and time until cure—doesn't exist in the same depth as information about posterior canal BPPV. It's impossible to estimate how many doctors are prescribing or using these treatments or which ones are used the most. Treatment of horizontal semicircular canal BPPV is relatively new and evolving. One of the five approaches has proved unsuccessful, but the four described in this chapter have sometimes succeeded, according to reports. Over time, these treatments may be modified or abandoned, and new ones may come along.

See below for an illustration pointing out the horizontal canal and its cupula. The semicircular canals are drawn out of proportion for the purposes of illustration in this figure and throughout the chapter.

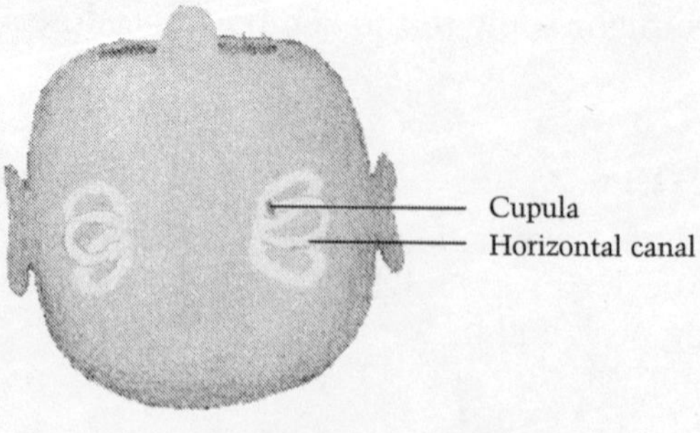

Figure 8-7: View of the head looking straight down from above.

How They Work

All four treatments consist of position changes intended to move debris from the horizontal semicircular canal into the utricle, where it won't cause further episodes of vertigo because the debris has re-attached, dissolved, broken down, or moved to where it can't cause symptoms. Most of these treatments are done by a health care professional (medical doctor, physical therapist, audiologist, occupational therapist, or possibly someone else). The exact method varies considerably from professional to professional.

The Procedures

If you are treated with the 270-degree positional maneuver also referred to as a "log roll" and described by Lempert and Tiel-Wilck (1996), it will consist of the following:

1. The practitioner will move you through a series of rapid head-position changes, 90 degrees at a time, toward the unaffected side, for a total of 270 degrees while you lie flat. (Your head will be moved quickly into each position and left there for 30 to 60 seconds.)
2. The practitioner will watch your eye movement to determine when to proceed to the next position.
3. If nystagmus persists, the procedure will be repeated.

The full contralateral roll (Figure 8-8) as described by Baloh in 1994 consists of the following:

1. The patient rolls through 360 degrees in four parts, toward the unaffected side, from flat on the back to flat on the back, 90 degrees per turn. Each position is held for one minute.
2. The overall procedure is repeated two to four times or until the nystagmus disappears.
3. Sometimes the patient is told to repeat the treatment at home.

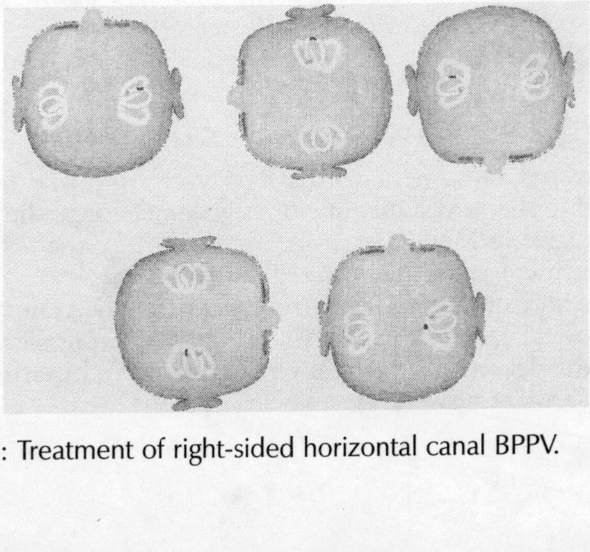

Figure 8-8: Treatment of right-sided horizontal canal BPPV.

If you have the liberatory maneuver as described by De la Meilleure, *et al.* (1996), you will experience the following:

1. You will lie flat on your back.
2. To induce nystagmus, the practitioner will lift your head 30 degrees from horizontal and turn you onto the side with the BPPV.
3. This position is maintained for five minutes with your head still flexed 30 degrees from the horizontal.
4. Observing your eyes for nystagmus, the practitioner will turn your head rapidly 180 degrees to the opposite side.
5. This position is maintained for five minutes. You will be told not to lie down or shake your head for 48 hours after the procedure.

The forced prolonged position maneuver described by Vannucchi, Giannoni, and Pagnini (1997) is uncomplicated. You lie on your back and roll onto your side opposite the ear with the horizontal canal BPPV. You maintain this side-lying position for 12 hours.

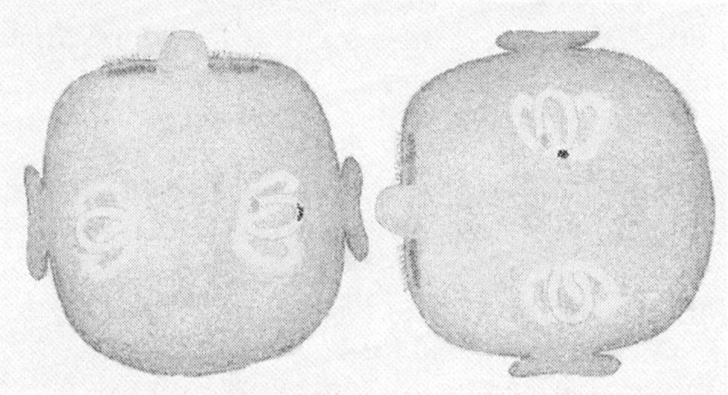

Figure 8-9: Prolonged position maneuver.

Success Rates

Just as with posterior BPPV, treatment maneuvers differ greatly as do the definitions of success and the methods for measuring it. Reports of success range from 50 to 90 percent. Numerous spontaneous remissions make score keeping difficult, according to reports.

Preventing Immediate Recurrence

Position and movement restrictions vary from one health-care professional to the next. Only one of these procedures, the liberatory maneuver of De le Meilleure, *et al.*, is thought by the originator to require movement restrictions after the procedure.

Because the horizontal canal is narrower than the posterior canal and is not the lowest canal when the head is upright, professionals generally think the debris will not easily return to it and that movement restrictions are not necessary.

Not for Everyone

The same limitations might apply to the horizontal canal treatments as to the CRP and Semont treatments (page 61-62.)

Possible Problems

Posterior canal BPPV may occur. If so, it can probably be treated successfully. Vertigo may occur during the procedure.

Possible Failure

These treatments might not work for any of the following reasons:

- The diagnosis is wrong.
- The wrong side is chosen.
- Not enough time is allowed for the debris to float out.
- Debris is stuck to the cupula and can't float out.
- The debris moves toward the cupula rather than into the utricle.

Further Options

If a procedure fails, it can be repeated or a new one tried. The diagnosis can also be re-checked.

References

Baloh, R.W. Reply to a letter by Lempert, "Horizontal Benign Positional Vertigo." *Neurology*, 44(11):2214, 1994.

Baloh, R.W., Jacobson, K., and Honrubia, V. "Horizontal Semicircular Canal Variant of Benign Positional Vertigo." *Neurology*, 43:2542-2549, 1993.

Brandt, T., and Daroff, R.B. "Physical Therapy for Benign Paroxysmal Positional Vertigo." *Archives of Otolaryngology-Head and Neck Surgery*, 106(8):484-485, 1980.

De la Meilleure, G., Dehaene, I., Depondt, M., Damman, W., Crevits, L., and Vanhooren, G. "Benign Paroxysmal Positional Vertigo of the Horizontal Canal." *Journal of Neurology, Neurosurgery, and Psychiatry*, 60(1):68-71, 1996.

Dornhoffer, J.L. and Colvin, G.B. "Benign Paroxysmal Positional Vertigo and Canalith Repositioning: Clinical Correlations." *American Journal of Otology*, 21:230-233, 2000.

Epley, J.M. "Canalith Repositioning Procedure," *Otolaryngology-Head and Neck Surgery*, 107(3):399-404, 1992.

Epley, J.R. "Benign Paroxysmal Positional Vertigo: New Methods of Diagnosis and Management." In Johnson, J.T., *et al., Instructional Courses*, Vol. 5, 197-207. St. Louis: Mosby Year Book, 1992.

Epley, J.M. "Caveats in Particle Repositioning for Treatment of Canalithiasis (BPPV)." *Operative Techniques in Otolaryngology-Head and Neck Surgery*, 8(2):68-76, 1997.

Fife, T.D. "Recognition and Management of Horizontal Canal Benign Positional Vertigo." *American Journal of Otology*, 19(3):345-351, 1998.

Herdman, S.J. "Physical Therapy in the Treatment of Patients with Benign Paroxysmal Positional Vertigo." *Neurology Report*, 20(3): 46-53, 1996.

Herdman, S.J. *Vestibular Rehabilitation*. Philadelphia: F.A. Davis Company, 1994.

Herdman, S.J. "Treatment of Benign Paroxysmal Positional Vertigo." *Physical Therapy*, 70(6):381-388, 1990.

Herdman, S., et al., "Single Treatment Approaches to BPPV." *Archives of Otolaryngology-Head and Neck Surgery*, 119:452, 1993.

Herdman, S.J. "Advances in the Treatment of Vestibular Disorders." *Physical Therapy*, 7(6):602-618, 1997.

Honrubia, V., et al. "Paroxysmal Positional Vertigo Syndrome." *American Journal of Otology*, 20:465-470, 1999.

Lempert, T., and Tiel-Wilck, K. "A Positional Maneuver for Treatment of Horizontal-Canal Benign Positional Vertigo." *Laryngoscope*, 106(4):476-478, 1996.

Lempert, T. "Horizontal Benign Positional Vertigo" (letter to the editor). *Neurology*, 44(11):2213-2214, 1994.

Nunez, R.A., Cass, S.P., and Furman, J.M. "Short- and Long-Term Outcomes of Canalith Repositioning for Benign Paroxysmal Positional Vertigo." *Otolaryngology-Head and Neck Surgery*, 122(5):647-652, 2000.

Nuti, D., Vannucchi, P., and Pagnini, P. "Benign Paroxysmal Positional Vertigo of the Horizontal-Canal Benign Positional Vertigo." *Journal of Vestibular Research*, 6(3):173-184, 1996.

Radtke, A. et al. "A Modified Epley's Procedure for Self-Treatment of Benign Paroxysmal Positional Vertigo." *Neurology*, 53: 1358-1360, 1999.

Steenerson, R.L., and Cronin, G.W. "Comparison of the Canalith Repositioning Procedure and Vestibular Habituation Training in Forty Patients with Benign Paroxysmal Positional Vertigo." *Otolaryngology-Head and Neck Surgery*, 114:61-64, 1996.

Vannucchi, P., Giannoni, B., and Pagnini, P. "Treatment of Horizontal Semicircular Canal Benign Paroxysmal Positional Vertigo." *Journal of Vestibular Research*, 7(1):1-6, 1997.

Welling, D.B., and Burnes, D.C., "The Incidence and Distribution of Cupular Deposits in the Labyrinth." *Laryngoscope*, 104:947, 1994.

Wolf, J.S., et al. "Success of the Modified Epley Maneuver in Treating Benign Paroxysmal Positional Vertigo." *Laryngoscope*, 109:900-903, 1999.

Chapter 9
Vestibular Rehabilitation

Additional symptoms and disturbances of balance function, beyond vertigo, can be significant problems for some people with BPPV, sometimes even after successful treatment of the positional vertigo. Vestibular rehabilitation is a therapy that may help relieve these symptoms.

Background, Goals

The term vestibular rehabilitation was coined in 1985 by two physical therapy researchers, Horak and Shumway-Cook, and is defined as "an exercise-based approach to managing and compensating for vestibular problems."

Vestibular rehabilitation aims to restore balance function to normal or as close to normal as possible and rid you of symptoms related to vestibular loss or malfunction. Via exercises, it attempts to:

- enable you to use vestibular information to the best of your ability for both balance and clear vision.
- use the proper combination of vestibular, visual, and proprioceptive information to maintain balance.
- learn to replace lost vestibular function.
- train your brain to adjust to altered messages from the inner ears.

Some other names for vestibular rehabilitation include vestibular physical therapy, vestibular PT, vestibular therapy, vestibular rehabilitation therapy, vestibular exercises, and VRT.

Physical therapy for vestibular problems is a relatively new concept. Doctors Cooksey and Cawthorne in the United Kingdom introduced systematic exercises for loss of vestibular function in 1944. In the U.S., these exercises were not widely embraced as a treatment for vestibular loss and dysfunction until much later. The first full-length book on vestibular rehabilitation, called *Vestibular Rehabilitation*, edited by S.J. Herdman, appeared in 1994. A second edition was published in 1999.

During the 1990s, the use of VRT increased significantly. Many physical therapy departments beginning to offer it along with their other services. Since it is relatively new, some therapists performing it are inexperienced, and some lack training.

Who Might Benefit

Vestibular rehabilitation may help reduce problems associated with any of the following:

- the presence of imbalance, unsteadiness, or visually-stimulated symptoms
- imbalance, unsteadiness, or visually-stimulated symptoms after successful medical or surgical treatment of BPPV
- residual or new symptoms and balance difficulties after BPPV surgery
- BPPV accompanied by a vestibular problem that has caused permanent loss of function
- stiff or weakened muscles or joints caused by avoiding certain movements and positions
- over-reliance on vision

Not only do many people with BPPV describe symptoms and balance problems in addition to episodes of positional vertigo, but computerized dynamic posturography studies have shown impaired balance. A study by Di Girolamo and others has shown that some people continue to have some degree of impairment even a month past the successful use of the Semont maneuver.

> "The results clearly show that, in BPPV patients, there is an impairment of the vestibular system, which seems unable to maintain a normal postural balance."
>
> — Di Girolamo, et al., *Acta Otolaryngologica*, 1998

How It Is Done

A physical or occupational therapist, with additional training in vestibular disorders and their treatment, usually provides vestibular rehabilitation. In some clinics and doctors' offices, an audiologist, registered nurse, or sometimes an unlicensed person supervised by a physician might provide therapy.

Generally speaking, health-care professionals trained in vestibular function and disorders will use exercises customized to fit each particular patient. Generic exercises that are the same from patient to patient continue to be suggested by some physicians and therapists but are felt by the majority of experts in the field to be of much less benefit than a customized program.

The Customized Program

The customized program begins with an assessment to determine your symptoms and functional limitations. This assessment may include:

- a questionnaire about current symptoms and their effect on you
- positional testing
- a battery of positioning and movement tests
- muscle performance testing
- tests of the range of motion of your joints
- eye movement testing

A health professional or health-care worker uses data from the assessment to design your exercise program, teaches you about the exercises and how and when to do them at home. Follow-up appointments may include further assessment as well as instructions for additional exercises. Below are examples of assessment findings and exercises that might be suggested. These are only three of many possible exercises.

- Muscle weakness—Undertake general conditioning program to strengthen muscles.
- Under-use of vestibular information and over-use of vision and proprioception—Stand barefooted on thick foam with eyes open, and stand in corner with eyes closed. Once these are mastered, stand barefooted on thick foam with eyes closed.
- Difficulty focusing on an object—Tape business card to wall at eye level. Stand just far enough away from card to be able to read it while moving head. With eyes focused on lettering, move head slowly from side to side.

Generic Exercises

The generic approach instructs everyone, regardless of his or her particular symptoms and problems, to do the same exercises. The Cawthorne-Cooksey exercises (Table 9-1) are probably the best known example of these pre-set lists. This approach is generally considered by experts to be inferior to the tailored program approach.

When to Stop, Seek Help

The health care professional providing the exercise instructions should include information about when to stop the exercises. Keep in mind that vertigo is expected from these exercises. In general, you should check with your health care provider for further instructions if you experience any of the following:

- pain, numbness or tingling in the neck, back, head, shoulders, hips, or ears
- ear pressure when not doing the exercises
- onset of ear ringing or hearing loss

Table 9-1: Cawthorne-Cooksey Exercises
(The health-care provider determines the number of repetitions.)

I. Lying down

A. Eye movements, first slowly and then more quickly
   1. up and down
   2. from side to side
   3. focusing on finger while moving it from three feet away to one foot away from face

B. Head movements, first slowly, then more quickly, and later with eyes closed
   1. bending forward and backward
   2. turning from side to side

II. Sitting

A. Eye movements as in I-A
B. Head movements as in I-B
C. Shoulder shrugging and circling
D. Bending forward and picking up objects from the ground

III. Standing

A. Eye movements as in I-A
B. Head movements as in I-B
C. Shoulder shrugging/circling as in II-C
D. Changing from sitting to standing with eyes open and with eyes shut
E. Throwing a small ball from hand to hand (above eye level)
F. Throwing a ball from hand to hand under knee
G. Changing from sitting to standing, and turning around (360 degrees) in between

IV. Moving around

A. Circling around a center person and playing catch with a large ball
B. Walking across room with eyes open and then closed
C. Walking up and down slope with eyes open and then closed
D. Walking up and down steps with eyes open and then closed
E. Playing any game involving stooping or stretching and aiming such as bowling or basketball

Not for Everyone

Because these treatment approaches work by inducing positional vertigo, people unable or unwilling to bring on their positional vertigo are not good candidates. Also, you may be advised not to do the exercises if you have any of the following problems: perilymph fistula, detached retina (a structure inside the eye), hydrocephalus (or any other condition increasing the pressure in and around the brain), cervical arthrosis, vertebrovascular insufficiency, chronic neck or back problems, prior back or neck surgery, osteoporosis, esophageal reflux, or a recent head, neck, or back injury. In some cases, the exercises may be altered to take these other health conditions into account. If you experience pain, particularly of the neck and back, during the exercises, you may ask to stop the exercises to avoid injury.

Possible Problems

In addition to positional vertigo, the exercises can produce disequilibrium (sometimes constant) and nausea. These can be present throughout the day, particularly during the first few days of the exercises.

Definition: Disequilibrium is a vague sense of unsteadiness, imbalance, tilting, or bumping into things.

Possible Failure

The exercises might not work for any of the following reasons:

- The diagnosis was incorrect.
- The exercises were done improperly.
- The patient was unable to tolerate the symptoms brought on by the required position changes.

If you undertake either generic or customized vestibular rehabilitation, you might keep in mind the following words by Brian McCabe, M.D.:

> "Seek out your vertigo, and suffer it whenever you can. This means to stimulate it frequently. Only you can build the tolerance in your brain to overcome your symptoms. Consider it like building muscle strength. A muscle begins to grow in strength only when the exercise begins to hurt.
>
> "If your vertigo is related to certain head positions, seek repeatedly that head position to tolerance, remembering that each spell brings you closer to the last, each spell is 'money in the bank.'"

—*Laryngoscope*, 1978 (with permission from the publisher)

References

Black, F.O., and Nashner, L.M. "Vestibulo-Spinal Control Differs in Patients with Reduced Versus Distorted Vestibular Function." *Acta Otolaryngologica*, 406:110-114, 1984.

Di Girolamo, et al. "Postural Control in Benign Paroxysmal Positional Vertigo Before and After Recovery." *Acta Otolaryngologica (Stockh)*, 118(3):289-293, 1998.

Ford-Smith, C.D. "The Individualized Treatment of a Patient with Benign Paroxysmal Positional Vertigo." *Physical Therapy*, 77(8):848-855, 1997.

Herdman, S.J. "Physical Therapy in the Treatment of Patients with Benign Paroxysmal Positional Vertigo." *Neurology Report*, 20(3):46-53, 1996.

Herdman, S.J. *Vestibular Rehabilitation*. Philadelphia: F.A. Davis Company, 1994.

Herdman, S.J. "Advances in the Treatment of Vestibular Disorders." *Physical Therapy*, 77(6):602-618, 1997.

Luxon, L.M., and Davies, R.A. *Handbook of Vestibular Rehabilitation*. San Diego: Singular Publishing Group, 1997.

McCabe, B.F. "Labyrinthine Exercises in the Treatment of Diseases Characterized by Vertigo: Their Physiologic Basis and Methodology." *Laryngoscope*, 80(9):1429-1433, 1978.

Shepard, N.T., and Telian, S.A. *Practical Management of the Balance Disorder Patient*. San Diego: Singular Publishing Group, Inc., 1996.

Chapter 10

Surgery

As mentioned earlier, the majority of people with BPPV will never have inner ear surgery. They will either improve on their own or while undergoing one medical (non-surgical) treatment or another. Surgery is not the first choice for treating BPPV because:

- Most cases of BPPV resolve either spontaneously or with medical treatment.
- Surgery causes permanent changes.
- Surgery involves risk to hearing and balance structures and functions and to nearby structures.
- Surgery involves risks associated with general anesthesia and with surgery in general.
- Surgery is expensive. It costs a great deal more than doing nothing or trying a medical (non-surgical) treatment.

The following information may be helpful if you find yourself in the minority who may need to consider surgery.

Factors Your Doctor Considers

Physicians look at a number of different factors to determine if surgery would be an appropriate treatment option. These factors or considerations can be divided into three groups: patient, physician, and general.

Patient Factors

- symptoms, their frequency and severity
- inability to function
- length of time the symptoms have been present
- presence of another inner ear problem accompanying the BPPV
- test results
- degree of impairment
- amount of misery present
- possible involvement of both ears
- hearing status of both ears
- age
- general condition

Physician Factors

- what the doctor was taught in medical school and during residency training
- what his or her experiences with different treatments have been
- which treatments the doctor believes in or feels have been proven through research
- the doctor's skills and abilities

General Factors

- the risk/benefit ratio
- the availability of facilities

Note on risk/benefit ratio: When determining the appropriateness of a treatment, in consultation with your doctor you must examine the risks and the possible benefits. The chance of bad results and their severity must be weighed against the chance of positive results and their degree of benefit. A judgment based on this comparison comes down to one question, "Is the possible benefit worth exposure to the risks?"

Questions for Your Doctor

When considering surgery as a treatment option, take the time to ask questions of your doctor, such as:

- What are the alternatives to this surgery? (Make it clear that you want to know about all the alternatives available, not just those offered by your particular doctor or covered by your health insurance plan.)
- Have all the medical treatments been offered and tried?
- Could any diseases or conditions other than BPPV cause the symptoms?
- What are the risks of the surgery to your general health and to your inner ear (hearing and balance) and nearby anatomic structures?
- What is the average or usual result of the surgery in the patients he/she has operated on?
- What is the worst result that can occur from the surgery?
- How many surgeries like this has your doctor done, and how many resulted in complications?

When asking about surgical results, try to pin your doctor down on his or her statistics, not those published in the literature by someone else. This someone else might have different skills, different experiences, or access to different testing/surgical equipment.

Doctors use terms like "control of vertigo" or "improvement" when talking about the positive results of surgery and "rare" or "unlikely" when referring to the chance of complications. Do not assume you understand what the doctors mean by these terms unless they actually define them. Ask for their definitions. For example, a doctor in one conversation may say that BPPV is "fairly common" and in another conversation say hearing loss from BPPV surgery is "rare." Yet the chance of developing BPPV is 10 to 64 in 100,000, while the chance of a hearing loss from one type of BPPV surgery is 3 in 100.

Ask your doctor for the names of some people on whom he or she has performed the surgery.

Ask questions and make sure you understand the answers before making any surgery decisions.

Deciding About Surgery

You can make an informed decision about surgery by listening carefully to your doctor, asking questions like the ones above, possibly discussing this information with a trusted friend or relative, perhaps speaking to someone who has had the surgery, and thinking through all options and ramifications of the proposed procedure. Get a second opinion, particularly if you have any doubts about the first.

If it is practical, take someone with you to the doctor's office when discussing something this important. A friend or relative can help you with asking questions and with recording or remembering answers to those questions.

Think about and discuss all the information you have collected with a friend or family member. Ask yourself if the reasons given by your doctor for surgery seem logical. Give yourself time to reflect upon your reasoning and motivations in deciding for or against surgery. Ideally your decision should be based on a multitude of factors including your physical, social, emotional, and financial well being.

You can also write or call the Vestibular Disorders Association to get information about local support groups in your area and to find other people in your area who have similar problems. (See Chapter 16, "Where to Get More Information.") If you have a computer and e-mail access, you can join groups discussing inner ear problems on the Internet. Keep in mind when doing this that many people join these organizations because they have difficult problems; many people who could tell success stories have no need for a support group. If you are thinking about surgery, examine your reasons carefully. Ask yourself the following questions:

- Do you look upon surgery as a quick fix for your problems?
- Do you feel that surgery is a sure thing or always better than medical treatment(s)?
- Do you think things can't get any worse if you have surgery?

The three reasons above are not good reasons to have surgery for BPPV. Surgery is not an instant fix and can require weeks of healing and recuperation. If you were to develop a complication, you could end up with a different set of problems, including hearing loss. Surgery would seem to be a reasonable option if all of the following are true:

- You have tried and failed to improve with a number of medical treatments.
- The episodes of vertigo prevent you from being and feeling safe.
- They prevent you from engaging in social activities.
- They prevent you from taking care of yourself or others (children, spouse, or parents), and/or working.
- They create physical misery.
- BPPV is your only inner ear problem.

The Surgeries

Posterior Semicircular Canal Occlusion

The surgery performed most frequently for posterior canal BPPV in the U.S. is the posterior semicircular canal occlusion procedure, also referred to as the posterior semicircular canal plugging procedure, posterior semicircular canal partitioning or fenestration, and occlusion of the posterior semicircular canal. Its aim is to halt the episodes of vertigo by stopping the movement of endolymph within the posterior semicircular canal. If the endolymph can't move, neither floating debris nor the cupula (with adhering debris) can move. Without movement of endolymph, the vertigo can't occur. This surgery is usually done by plugging or occluding the canal with bone chips (and/or other materials), or by using a laser, or by using both laser and bone chips. Some physicians have their own variations of the surgery that might differ from the one described here.

How It Is Done

While you are under general anesthesia, your surgeon makes a C-shaped incision behind your ear, removes enough mastoid bone to locate the posterior semicircular canal, and creates a hole into the canal. During a bone chip procedure, enough chips are inserted to create a dam across the width of the canal. (See Figure 10-1.) During a laser procedure, your doctor uses a laser to create the dam (occlusion).

After the Surgery

As the ear heals, new bone growth occurs in the area containing the bone chips and creates a solid wall that prevents the endolymph

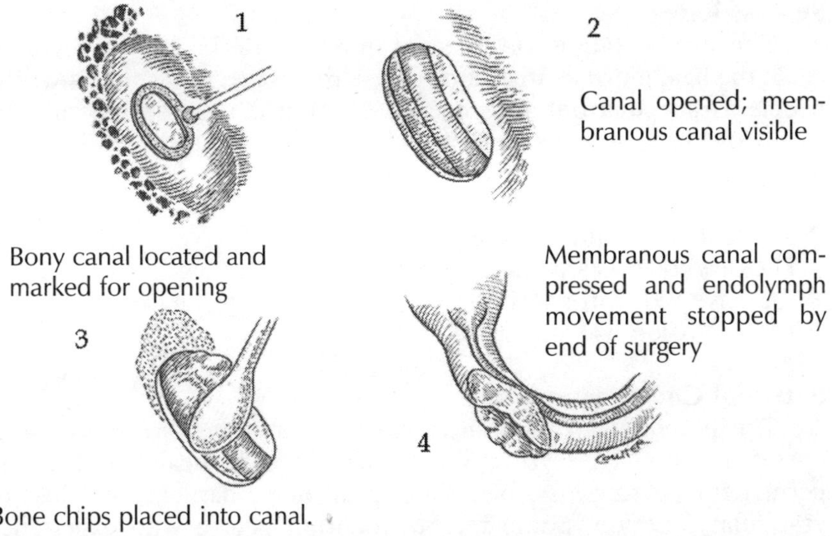

Figure 10-1: Posterior Semicircular Occlusion with Bone Chips. (From Hirsch, B.E. et al., "Translabyrinthine Approach to Skull Base Tumors with Hearing Preservation," *American Journal of Otology,* 14(6):533-543, 1993. Reprinted with permission.)

from moving. This surgery usually requires a hospital stay of two to five days. (One report in a medical journal described the procedure as same-day surgery.) Most people are back to work and their usual activities in six weeks or less. Older people generally require the most recuperation time.

If you have this surgery, your postoperative period may include:

- a hearing loss lasting from three to four weeks
- disequilibrium lasting from one week to several weeks, maybe even months
- motion sensitivity
- unsteadiness
- a feeling of motion when you press on the external ear or over the mastoid cavity (in the area of the incision)
- continued symptoms of BPPV for a week or somewhat more (until healing completes the occlusion)

Disequilibrium: Vague sense of unsteadiness, imbalance, tilting, or bumping into things that can occur in association with vestibular problems.

Vestibular rehabilitation therapy may also be suggested after the surgery.

Success Rates

The success rate is 100 percent in nearly all the studies reported on in medical journals including one with long-term results in which people as far out from surgery as 199 months were still symptom-free. However, some people not included in these studies have failed to improve with surgery.

Possible Reasons for Failure

- The diagnosis was wrong.
- You have BPPV in another canal or the opposite ear.
- The occlusion was incomplete.

Potential Complications

The potential for complications exist anytime the inner ear is operated upon. These complications include surgical labyrinthitis, permanent hearing loss, infection, facial nerve damage, and loss of vestibular function. Some reports mention people who experience long-term disequilibrium after the surgery. General anesthesia can also result in complications, although a serious complication from anesthesia is rare in otherwise healthy individuals.

Singular Neurectomy

A surgery done only occasionally in the U.S. is the singular neurectomy, also called the posterior ampullary nerve transection, singular nerve section, or transection of the singular nerve. The goal of this surgery is to stop abnormal balance information from a posterior semicircular canal from reaching the brain and causing vertigo. To accomplish this, a surgeon cuts the nerve that carries this information. The nerve in question (a branch of the vestibular nerve) is referred to as the singular nerve or sometimes the posterior ampullary nerve, hence the name(s) of the surgery.

While you are under local anesthesia, your surgeon makes an incision inside your external auditory canal around the tympanic membrane and enters your middle ear. The surgeon locates a specific area of the middle ear, makes an opening, drills through bone covering the nerve, and cuts the nerve. Some surgeons perform this surgery after making a C- shaped incision behind the ear.

In depth (anesthesia):

General anesthesia: You are given gas or intravenous drugs to cause and maintain a complete loss of consciousness. Usually you will have a tube down your throat so the anesthesiologist can "breathe for you" while you are unable to breathe on your own.

Regional anesthesia: An anesthetic is injected near a large col-

lection of nerves or the spinal canal to "numb" a large area such as an arm or everything from the waist down.
Local anesthesia: An anesthetic agent is injected directly into the area in need of "deadening" such as a cut requiring stitches.
Topical anesthesia: An anesthetic agent is sprayed, poured, or rubbed onto an area in need of numbing such as the tympanic membrane.

This procedure is not performed often because it is technically demanding. The nerve can be difficult or impossible to find and cut, and some people sustain permanent hearing loss.

After the Surgery

The hospital stay for this surgery can be two to four days with a return to work in two to three weeks. A mild sense of unsteadiness and nystagmus may be present for a couple of days after the surgery.

Success Rates

Three studies reported success rates of 97 percent, 69 percent, and 88 percent.

Possible Reasons for Failure

- wrong diagnosis
- BPPV in another canal of the same ear or a canal of the opposite ear
- failure to locate and cut the singular nerve

Potential Complications

The potential exists for complications anytime the ear is operated upon. These complications include permanent hearing loss, surgical labyrinthitis, infection, facial nerve damage, and loss of vestibular function. Hearing loss is the complication most commonly reported in medical journals. General anesthesia, when used, can also result in complications, although serious complications from anesthesia are rare.

Other Surgery

One physician has reported on another surgery, utricular macular ablation, specifically developed for posterior canal BPPV. This is a laser procedure that destroys the macula of the utricle, thereby eliminating the otoconia. The theory behind this surgery is that loose otoconia cause BPPV and that destroying them will stop more debris from entering the posterior semicircular canal and causing BPPV.

One further note: In some cases, people with BPPV accompanied by other inner ear disorders may be offered other surgical options specific to their case. Information about other surgeries, such as labyrinthectomy and vestibular nerve section, for vestibular disorders is available in other publications of the Vestibular Disorders Association.

References

Anthony, P.F. "Utricular Macular Ablation for Benign Paroxysmal Positional Vertigo." *Ear Nose and Throat Journal*, 75(7):416-421, 1996.

Antonelli, P.J., et al. "Mechanical Versus CO_2 Laser Occlusion of the Posterior Semicircular Canal in Humans." *American Journal of Otology*, 17:416-420, 1996.

Baloh, R.W., and Honrubia, V. Clinical *Neurophysiology of the Vestibular System*. Philadelphia: F.A. Davis Company, 1990.

Dingle, A.F., Hawthorne, M.R., and Kumar, B.U. "Fenestration and Occlusion of the Posterior Semicircular Canal, for Benign Positional Vertigo." *Clinical Otolaryngology*, 17:300-302, 1992.

Fernandes, C.M. "Singular Neurectomy in South African Practice." *South African Journal of Surgery*, 31(2):79-80, 1993.

Furman, J.M., and Cass, S.P. *Balance Disorders: A Case-Study Approach*. Philadelphia: F.A. Davis, 1996.

Gacek, R.R. "Technique and Results of Singular Neurectomy for the Management of Benign Paroxysmal Positional Vertigo." *Acta Otolaryngologica (Stockh)*, 115(2):154-157, 1995.

Gacek, R.R., and Gacek, M.R. "Singular Neurectomy in the Management of Paroxysmal Positional Vertigo." *Otolaryngologic Clinics of North America*, 27(2):363-379, 1994.

Gacek, R.R. "Further Observations on Posterior Ampullary Nerve Transection for Positional Vertigo." *Annals of Otology, Rhinology and Laryngology*, 87(3 Pt 1):300-305, 1978.

Glasscock, M.E., and Shambaugh, G.E. *Surgery of the Ear*. Fourth edition. Philadelphia: W.B. Saunders Company, 1990.

Hawthorne, M., and El-Naggar, M. "Fenestration and Occlusion of Posterior Semicircular Canal for Patients with Intractable Benign Paroxysmal Positional Vertigo." *The Journal of Laryngology and Otology*, 108:935-939, 1994.

Kartush, J.M., and Sargent, E.W. "Posterior Semicircular Canal Occlusion for Benign Paroxysmal Positional Vertigo - CO_2 Laser-Assisted Technique: Preliminary Results." *Laryngoscope*, 105:268-274, 1995.

Meyerhoff, W.L. "Surgical Section of the Posterior Ampullary Nerve." *Laryngoscope*, 95(8):933-5, 1985.

Pace-Balzan, A., and Rutka, J.A. "Non-Ampullary Plugging of the Posterior Semicircular Canal for Benign Paroxysmal Positional Vertigo." *Journal of Laryngology and Otology*, 105:901-906, 1991.

Parnes, L.S. "Update on Posterior Canal Occlusion for Benign Paroxysmal Positional Vertigo." *Otolaryngologic Clinics of North America*, 29(2):333-342, 1996.

Parnes, L.S., and McClure, J.A. "Posterior Semicircular Canal Occlusion in the Normal Hearing Ear." *Otolaryngology-Head and Neck Surgery*, 104(1):52-57, 1991.

Pulec, J.L. "Ablation of Posterior Semicircular Canal for Benign Paroxysmal Positional Vertigo." *Ear, Nose, and Throat Journal*, 76(1):17-22, 1997.

Silverstein, H., and White, D.W. "Wide Surgical Exposure for Singular Neurectomy in the Treatment of Benign Positional Vertigo." *Laryngoscope*, 100(7):701-6, 1990.

Suzuki, M., Kadir, A., Takamoto, M., and Hayashi, N. "Experimental Model of Vertigo Induced by Detached Otoconia." *Acta Otolaryngologica (Stockh)*, 116(2):269-72, 1996.

Walsh, R.M., et al. "Long-Term Results of Posterior Semicircular Canal Occlusion for Intractable Benign Paroxysmal Positional Vertigo." *Clinical Otolaryngology*, 24:316-323, 1999.

Zappia, J.J. "Posterior Semicircular Canal Occlusion for Benign Paroxysmal Positional Vertigo." *American Journal of Otology*, 17:749-754, 1996.

Chapter 11

Prognosis

When an individual case of BPPV has just begun, it is difficult to accurately predict its course. However, statistics compiled by physicians and others provide general clues about outcomes in various situations and with different treatments, as follows:

- Only about 1 percent of people diagnosed with BPPV uncomplicated by other problems will require surgery to rid themselves of disabling symptoms.
- BPPV unaccompanied by other vestibular disorders is not usually considered progressive and causes no proven permanent damage to vestibular function or hearing. Some people with BPPV unaccompanied by other vestibular disorders become more symptomatic over time, but this is not the general pattern.

Note: Some conditions that result in BPPV, such as occlusion of the anterior vestibular artery, can cause permanent damage and symptoms of which BPPV is only one.

- Posterior canal BPPV in one ear only, unaccompanied by any other inner ear conditions, has the highest chance of spontaneous remission or successful treatment.
- It's generally thought that many cases of BPPV will go away without treatment. One study suggests an 80 percent rate of spontaneous remission. However, few recent studies assess the percentage of people getting well without treatment.
- A significant number of people with BPPV have the symptoms on and off for years.
- Some experts feel that BPPV resulting from head injury or ear surgery will last only weeks to months and that BPPV accompanying ear infection, degeneration related to age, vascular occlusion, or Meniere's disease has a greater chance of becoming persistent.

Note: Meniere's disease may cause permanent damage to the utricle, which may lead to a more persistent form of BPPV.

- The chance of BPPV occurring in both ears is low. It has been estimated that 10 percent of people with BPPV unaccompanied by any other inner ear problems will probably develop it in both ears and that 20 percent of people with post-traumatic BPPV will have problems in both ears.

- When BPPV occurs in more than one ear or more than one canal, the chance of successful treatment decreases.
- No statistics exist about time lost from work because of BPPV or the number of people disabled by BPPV, but both are generally thought to be low.

Prognosis after Treatment

Posterior Canal

"The success rate of CRP varies among practitioners, but it is generally accepted that CRP offers an immediate relief of BPPV in a majority of patients."

—Honrubia, *et al., American Journal of Otology*, 1999.

Of those people having canalith repositioning, most studies suggest a 90 percent or better rate of success after the first sequence of one, two, or three treatments one week apart. Studies also suggest that the rate of recurrence after successful treatment can be as high as 32 to 45 percent. One study found that of the people having one recurrence, 22 percent would have multiple recurrences. Dornhoffer and Colvin found a 50 percent recurrence rate in people who also had Meniere's disease.

If you undergo CRP, odds are excellent that your immediate symptoms will stop. However, you face up to 45 percent odds that the symptoms will return at some point. If they do return, odds are perhaps 20 percent that they will return more than once. Some clinics teach self-treatment techniques to people prone to recurrences. If you fall into this category, ask your doctor if self-treatment is appropriate for your situation.

Anterior Canal Variant

Few statistics are available for this variant. Honrubia, et al., reported a success rate of 50 percent in treating this variant with the CRP. The recurrence rate is unknown.

Horizontal Canal Variant

The horizontal canal variant of BPPV was only identified as an entity in 1985 and does not occur frequently. This makes information less readily available than for the posterior canal variety.

In one U.S. study of 13 cases, Baloh and colleagues found that six had one bout of horizontal BPPV lasting from three days to five weeks and the remaining seven had recurring bouts over the next two to 20 years when untreated. Vannucchi and colleagues, in Italy, found that a group of 15 people receiving no treatment had their symptoms resolve in 19 to 60 days.

Honrubia and others found that people treated for canalithiasis of the horizontal canal had a 33 percent rate of cure, and those treated for cupulolithiasis had a 50 percent cure rate, at the UCLA clinic. The rate of recurrence is not known.

References

Baloh, R.W., Jacobson, K., and Honrubia, V. "Horizontal Semicircular Canal Variant of Benign Positional Vertigo." *Neurology*, 43:2542-2549, 1993.

De la Meilleure, et al. "Benign Paroxysmal Positional Vertigo of the Horizontal Canal," *Journal of Neurology, Neurosurgery, and Psychiatry*, 60(1):68-71, 1996.

Furman, J.M., and Cass, S.P. *Balance Disorders: A Case-Study Approach*. Philadelphia: F.A. Davis, Company, 1996.

Gross, E.M., et al. "Intractable Benign Paroxysmal Positional Vertigo in Patients with Meniere's Disease." *Laryngoscope*, 110:655-659, 2000.

Herdman, S.J. *Vestibular Rehabilitation*. Second edition. Philadelphia: F.A. Davis Company, 1999.

Honrubia, V., et al. "Paroxysmal Positional Vertigo Syndrome." American Journal of Otology, 20:465-470, 1999.

Nunez, R.A., Cass, S.P., and Furman, J.M. "Short and Long-Term Outcomes of Canalith Repositioning for Benign Paroxysmal Positional Vertigo." *Otolaryngology-Head and Neck Surgery*, 122(5):647-652, 2000.

Schuknecht, H.F. "Cupulolithiasis." *Archives of Otolaryngology-Head and Neck Surgery*, 90:765-778, 1969.

Vannucchi, P., Giannoni, B., and Pagnini, P. "Treatment of Horizontal Semicircular Canal Benign Paroxysmal Positional Vertigo." *Journal of Vestibular Research*, 7(1)1-6, 1997.

Chapter 12
Coping

How does someone cope with BPPV? People with mild types of BPPV should not have to cope for long. Either the problem will stop with treatment, or it will stop on its own in weeks to months. If you have only begun to experience BPPV, it will most likely be limited to short bursts of vertigo in certain positions, and chances are you'll be back to normal shortly. If you have had BPPV for a longer time and/or have one of the more severe forms, information in addition to that covered in this chapter can be found in Appendix E: More Coping Tips.

Most short-term coping revolves around activities meant to stop the BPPV, stay safe, and maintain a sense of well being.

Stopping the BPPV

The most important first step in stopping BPPV is to find a physician trained and experienced in vestibular disorders. (See Chapter 13: "Who's Who in Otologic Health Care.") Find out from this health care provider what you should do to stop the BPPV and to stay safe. Under certain circumstances, your provider may tell you to avoid movements that provoke your symptoms; under other circumstances you may be advised to move in ways meant to provoke symptoms en route to making them go away. Formulate a plan with your health care provider and try to stick with the approach you decide upon, and use advice from other people only if it fits the plan. If you can't or won't follow the plan, tell your health care provider so he or she can perhaps find another provider or another plan better suited to your needs.

Staying Safe

Constantly thinking about your positional vertigo is not a good idea; however, it's wise to identify safety concerns and to address them. This means asking your doctor about the safety of yourself and others when you work, drive, climb ladders, bicycle, swim, run, or engage in other activities. If you have to decide on your own what activities are safe or how to make your activities safer, you should consider:

- head positions that cause problems
- the severity of your vertigo
- what types of symptoms you might have between episodes of positional vertigo
- whether you have become more dependent upon vision or proprioception than normal
- head positions and movements necessary at work
- activities that interest you, including requirements and location

Your doctor will not be able to make every decision for you about safety concerns. Only you know how well or poorly you are feeling, what your capabilities have been, and what level of confidence you have in your present abilities.

Some specific activities with safety considerations you need to consider include driving, piloting, swimming, and boating.

Driving

No clear universal rules cover whether or not a person with BPPV should be driving an automobile. Government rules dealing with fitness to drive differ from state to state, province to province, and country to country. For example, the Canadian Medical Association publishes a *Physician Guide to Driver Examination* that includes a passage relevant to BPPV:

> "Patients with temporary vestibular conditions such as acute labyrinthitis or positional vertigo should be advised not to drive until the condition has subsided or responded to treatment."

Check the driving rules of your state, province, or country, and consult your doctor before getting behind the wheel. In 1997 the American Neurotological Society recommended that its physician members advise patients with BPPV to use discretion when deciding about their ability to drive safely.

> "Although some patients who experience dizziness can drive a car safely when symptoms are mild, do so at your own risk. Nothing I say or write in the chart, no medication, can take away your legal responsibility if you are involved in an accident."
>
> —G. Hughes, M.D., *American Journal of Otology*, 1990

If your doctor advises you to not drive, follow the advice. The decision to drive, particularly in areas with large populations and busy roads, should not be taken lightly. As you make your personal decision, put safety first.

Piloting an Aircraft

For piloting an aircraft, fewer gray areas exist than for driving, and only one agency regulates the skies above the entire U.S., the Federal Aviation Agency (FAA). Its regulations concerning first-, second-, and third-class aviators include requirements for medical certification. One of these denies certification to an aviator with a "disease or condition manifested by, or that may reasonably be expected to be manifested by, vertigo or a disturbance of equilibrium."

It follows from this requirement that someone with BPPV should not be piloting an aircraft and cannot be medically cleared to fly in the U.S. even if currently licensed.

Swimming and Boating

If you have BPPV, swimming or boating might cause life-threatening problems under circumstances that cause you to lose your bearings.

> "Also, avoid swimming. Under water you can become disoriented and not know which way is up."
>
> —G. Hughes, M.D., *American Journal of Otology*, 1990

If you feel ill or drowsy, don't skipper a boat or jet ski. When traveling on small pleasure craft, wear a securely fastened flotation device approved by the Coast Guard. If you fall or are knocked overboard, you will float with your head held out of the water if you are wearing a vest. While moving about on a boat, keep both feet on the deck and at least one hand on a railing, seat, or other object firmly attached to the deck.

Well Being

Some people with BPPV may experience fear, loss of confidence, and other feelings that undermine their sense of well being. Considering how much disruption and chaos BPPV can cause, this is understandable.

When you feel afraid, try to determine exactly what you fear. If you can identify the fear precisely, you may be able to lessen it. For example, if you fear that people will find out about your problem, it might be best to take them aside and tell them about it.

> "I gradually felt better, began socializing more and began telling people about my condition. I felt better having them

know why I couldn't read or why I couldn't ride with them unless they drove like a 'Sunday driver.'"

—S.L., Wisconsin, letter to the author, 1999

"The worst part has been regaining my confidence that if the highway is rough I will not become dizzy. Every month is better as I continue to try new-old things and find that I do not have any problems."

—C.K., *More Stories and Strategies*, 1999

Coping with Advice

Coping also may include listening to advice and suggestions on how to avoid positional vertigo and how to treat BPPV from various people. Much of this information will be based on personal experiences or common sense. Unfortunately, while the advice might be good in some cases, in others it might only be partly good and in others not good at all. Think carefully before acting upon such advice from people other than health care professionals. Since BPPV varies from case to case, not all advice is universally helpful. Indeed, advice based on personal experience is often contradictory, as the following examples show:

"Sleep on the affected side."

—S.L., Wisconsin, letter to the author, 1999

"A friend of mine told me not to sleep on the affected side. This was the best piece of advice I received from anyone. It made a huge difference in how severe my symptoms were."

—V.N., Pennsylvania, letter to the author, 1999

Summary

The amount and type of coping with BPPV usually depends upon the type of BPPV present. People with the milder varieties will not need to cope much or for long. Those with the more severe varieties might need more help with coping. Appendix E contains further tips for people with severe types of BPPV.

References

______. Vestibular Disorders Association. *More Stories and Strategies*, 1995.

Baloh, R.W., and Halmagyi, G.M. *Disorders of the Vestibular System*. New York: Oxford University Press, 1996.

Federal Aviation Administration. "Federal Aviation Regulations." http://www.safetydata.com/far-67.htm. Oct. 30, 1997.

Hughes, G.B. "Paroxysmal Positional Vertigo: What the Patient Needs to Know." *American Journal of Otology*, 11(5):306, 1990.

Chapter 13

Who's Who in Otologic Health Care

If you seek treatment for your BPPV, you will want to find a doctor with the right kind of training and experience. Along the way, you may encounter health professionals with varied titles, duties, and functions. This chapter will describe many types of physicians and other professionals such as physical therapists and nurses and explain:

- who they are
- what they do
- what you should expect from them
- what their titles mean
- how much education and training they have had

Note on licensing and/or certification testing: Holding a state license in medicine, nursing, physical therapy, audiology, occupational therapy, or anything else does not guarantee quality. However, dealing only with health care workers who are licensed is one way for you to know they have met minimum requirements such as schooling and passing a test. If a state board determines that someone should stop practicing in a health care profession, he or she will not be able to get work in that profession anywhere in the U.S.

Doctors

General Expectations

Generally, you can expect a doctor and his or her office staff to:

- treat you with dignity and courtesy.
- include you in all aspects of your care.
- record your medical history and your current situation.
- examine you.
- select pertinent tests and interpret their results.
- diagnose your problem.
- give you information about the diagnosis and what you need to do.
- discuss all treatment options available.

- refer to another appropriate specialist or clinic if unable to diagnose or treat your problem.
- explain all testing and treatment ahead of time.
- keep accurate written documentation of your condition.
- schedule a follow-up appointment after treatment is started to assess its impact.
- maintain confidentiality of all medical information (However, when you have signed the release most health insurance companies insist upon, your information will be shared with them as they require).

Medical Education

The education of medical students in the U.S. differs somewhat from school to school, but in general these students spend their first two years in classrooms studying science and learning some of the skills needed to examine and treat people. Anatomy and physiology, including perhaps one lecture about the ear, are covered during this time.

The second two years are spent among patients in hospitals, clinics, and doctors' offices. During this two-year period, every student gains experience in some areas of medicine but not in others unless he or she specifically chooses to study it. Otolaryngology-head and neck surgery is one of the areas of study not required by all medical schools. Those that do require it may schedule as little as one week of study for otolaryngology.

The average medical student receives an extremely limited introduction to the inner ear. Because of this, you may meet practicing physicians who have virtually no knowledge of BPPV or the working of the vestibular system.

M.D. Licensing

In the U.S., all doctors must be licensed to practice medicine by the state they work in. (Two exceptions are the Veterans Administration health system and the military. Doctors for these entities need only be licensed in some U.S. state, not necessarily the one in which they are working.) The license verifies that a physician has graduated from an accredited school of medicine and has passed a standardized test showing at least minimum competence. It does not indicate that the doctor has received specialty training. The Board of Medicine or agency with a similar title in each state regulates medical licensing.

Neither M.D. licensing nor advanced certification guarantees in-depth knowledge of the inner ear, particularly vestibular function.

Specialists

The categories below include the kinds of physicians who might be experienced in treating BPPV.

Otolaryngologist-Head and Neck Surgeon

The general medical specialty that includes matters related to the ear is otolaryngology-head and neck surgery. An otolaryngologist-head and neck surgeon is a medical doctor who specializes in disorders of the head and neck, especially those related to the ear, nose, and throat. This doctor may also be referred to as an otolaryngologist, otorhinolaryngologist, ear-nose-throat (ENT) doctor, or ENT specialist.

Otolaryngologists don't just specialize in problems of the ear; they do a large assortment of things such as surgery for cancer of the mouth, tongue, throat, or voice box, and plastic surgery for problems such as cleft lips or palates. They treat nosebleeds, nose fractures, and middle ear infections. They remove tonsils and adenoids, perform sinus surgery, and might do allergy work.

Their academic education includes four years of college and four years of medical school. However, these first eight years of higher education might include only extremely limited exposure to inner ear anatomy/physiology and diseases.

Post-medical school training, also called "residency training," in this specialty has a large surgical focus and lasts for at least five years; only a small portion of this is dedicated specifically to otology. After their training is completed, they are eligible to take a certification test known as a "board" given by the American Academy of Otolaryngology. Once they pass the examination, they can refer to themselves as "board certified" and use the title of Fellow of the American College of Surgeons (F.A.C.S.). (Fellow, in this context, means "member.")

If a doctor is "board eligible," it means he or she has completed the required years of residency training but has not taken the certification examination or has not passed it.

In depth (board certification test): The purpose of this test is to provide assurance to the public that a physician specialist certified by a member board of the American Board of Medical Specialties (ABMS) has successfully completed an approved educational program and an evaluation process. This includes an examination designed to assess the knowledge, skills, and experience required for high-quality patient care in that specialty.

Otologist/Neurotologist

This is an M.D. who has completed a residency in otolaryngology and studied otology/neurotology for a year or two as an otology or neurotology fellow in a program certified by the American Board of Otology in the sub-specialty of Otology/Neurotology.

Some physicians who have not completed any further training beyond the basic residency use the title otologist or neurotologist or describe themselves as practicing otology or neurotology. They may or may not have expert knowledge about BPPV. Ask the office before making an appointment to verify that the physician completed a fellowship in otology or neurotology. Only a physician who has completed the otology/neurotology fellowship in a certified program can state that he or she is certified as an otologist or neurotologist.

Note: A study done in 1997 questioned members of the American Neurotology Society about the fraction of their practice dedicated to neurotology. Questionnaires were completed by about 70 percent of the 402 members in the U.S. and Canada. Of these, about 90 percent called themselves a "vestibular regional authority." Even so, about half spent less than 30 percent of their time with people having a vestibular problem. Only 8 percent spent 81 to 100 percent of their time on vestibular medicine. If this ratio held true for the remainder of the membership who did not respond to the survey, it would mean that as few as 32 neurotologists in the U.S. and Canada devote their practice nearly exclusively to neurotology.

Neurologist

A neurologist is a medical doctor who has undergone four years of residency training in medical problems of the brain, nervous system, and nerves. Neurologists' treatments don't include surgery.

A neurologist may become your primary physician for BPPV or may be used only to help rule out neurological causes of your problem. Many neurological problems can cause dizziness, lightheadedness, and vertigo.

Neurologists that specialize in conditions related to BPPV may call themselves neurotologists, otoneurologists, or otolaryngic neurologists. Only a small number of neurologists are trained and experienced in BPPV.

In depth (choosing a doctor): Choosing a doctor to treat your BPPV can be a complicated affair. You may have many specialists to choose from as well as all the insurance rules, geographic considerations, institutional policies, and your own personal preferences to sort through.

In a perfect world, you might see someone with a practice limited to treating people with BPPV. In the real world, you will see someone with a varied practice that includes cases of BPPV. If you have BPPV and co-existing vestibular problems, or if previous treatment for BPPV has not worked, consider making the effort to find a physician whose practice is limited to neurotology.

The majority of insurance policies will limit your choice of physician in some way. You need to check your policy manual or call the insurance company to be certain you are following its rules and policies. If you belong to an HMO or other managed care insurance organization, you will be sent to someone under contract to the organization. The contract is not necessarily made with the best doctor; sometimes it is made with the doctor who accepts the least amount of money from the HMO. This, in and of itself, does not mean the doctor under contract is in any way inferior. Remember that you can go to anyone you want if you are able and willing to pay for it yourself.

If you prefer a certain hospital, select a doctor on the medical staff at that hospital. You can get information about this by calling a doctor's office and asking. Also, some hospitals have ask-a-nurse and other call-in programs that give the names of their physicians.

You must decide what you think makes a "good" doctor. Is it someone who is efficient and business-like? One who spends a great deal of time with you? Is it a doctor fresh from residency training with new ideas and methods or perhaps an older doctor with a lot of experience? Is it someone who says "don't worry" or someone who tells you everything? Do you care only about technical expertise, or is "bedside manner" also important? Decide what you prize most highly before you begin to look.

The best place to start, if you will be doing the selection, is your family doctor. Ask for his or her recommendation. Find out if your doctor has sent others with your problem to this doctor and if the outcomes were good.

You can also ask friends, relatives, and neighbors if they know of a doctor. If you know any health care professionals socially, ask for their thoughts on the matter. You can get state-by-state flyers from the Vestibular Disorders Association (VEDA) that list doctors interested in vestibular disorders. If you are a VEDA member, you can also ask other members for advice via the VEDA pen pal lists, called Link Lists. Also, look for the Dizzinews mailing list on the Internet. (See Chapter 16, "Where to Get More Information" for mailing list instructions.)

In depth (malpractice and competence): If you're concerned about the number of lawsuits involving a prospective doctor, you may be able to review complaints and other problems through the agency that regulates medical practice in your state. The State of Florida, for example, has such information available on the

Internet. Also, a book called *Questionable Doctors* lists doctors that its authors feel may not practice safely.

If a health care professional has settled a malpractice claim out of court, it does not automatically mean the professional did anything wrong. For example, settlement may occur because the doctor's insurance company does not want to pay for a jury trial. Most malpractice insurance policies have a clause forcing the insured to settle out of court at the whim of the insurance company. If the insured does not comply, he or she loses insurance coverage.

Keep in mind that to find someone responsible in a malpractice case, the jury does not need to be unanimous and does not have to be convinced beyond a reasonable doubt. It only has to be sure by a preponderance (more than half) of the evidence. A lot of room is left for error.

Other MDs

Radiologist

A radiologist is a doctor specializing in the reading of X-rays and other body imaging such as CT or CAT scans and MRIs. If you must have X-rays, you will most likely not meet or see the radiologist, but you will receive a bill for his or her services. A technician will actually do the test.

Optometrist

An optometrist is not an M.D. but has completed four years of undergraduate college and is also a graduate of a college of optometry. Optometrists can examine eyes and prescribe glasses and medicines. They don't usually have any training or knowledge about BPPV or any other vestibular disorder.

Ophthalmologist

An ophthalmologist is an M.D. specializing in diseases and surgery of the eyes. Ophthalmologists don't usually have much knowledge of BPPV or any other vestibular problem.

Neuro-Ophthalmologist

A neuro-ophthalmologist is an M.D. who specializes in neurological vision changes. These specialists generally have no training in vestibular disorders. If you are sent to a neuro-ophthalmologist for treatment of BPPV, ask carefully about the training and experience qualifying him or her to treat a vestibular disorder.

Associated Professionals

Audiologist

According to the American Speech-Language-Hearing Association (ASHA), audiologists are hearing health care professionals who specialize in prevention, identification, and assessment of hearing disorders and provide treatment and rehabilitative services.

An audiologist with full credentials can only begin to practice once he or she has completed five to six years of college with a bachelor's and master's degree (or a Ph.D.) in audiology, has spent nine months in supervised practice, and has passed a nationally administered examination. At that point audiologists can use the title Certificate of Clinical Competence in Audiology, abbreviated CCC-A. Most states require licensing and fulfillment of requirements similar to those for the CCC-A for someone to practice audiology.

Audiologists' education and training prepares them to test hearing, administer many different vestibular tests, dispense hearing aids and provide other hearing services and treatments. If you have questions about hearing tests, hearing aids, and other hearing treatments, the audiologist in your doctor's office may be able to answer them.

Physical Therapist

Some symptoms associated with BPPV may make it hard or impossible for you to perform routine tasks. People having any medical or surgical procedure that results in complete loss of vestibular function in one or both ears may have significant symptoms that interfere with their daily routines. Individuals in these situations may be sent to a physical therapist (PT or RPT) and/or an occupational therapist (OT or OTR) for evaluation and treatment.

According to the American Physical Therapy Association, a physical therapist is able to evaluate your joint motion, muscle strength and endurance, functional ability, muscle tone and reflexes, appearance and stability of walking, integrity of sensation and perception, and your performance of daily living activities and developmental activities. Physical therapy techniques include therapeutic exercise, joint mobilization and range-of-motion exercises, relaxation exercises, therapeutic massage, biofeedback, training in the activities of daily living, and ambulation (walking) training.

These therapists enter their profession after completing at least a four-year college course, and many start with a master's degree. They must take and pass a national exam and meet any other requirements of the state board regulating the practice of physical therapists in their state before they can use the title of Registered Physical Therapist (RPT).

Therapists who have had additional training and experience can assess balance, abnormal eye movements, and reactions to position change. They can teach you exercises (vestibular rehabilitation) to accustom your brain to new vestibular signals and can also perform canalith repositioning. However, both canalith repositioning and vestibular rehabilitation are somewhat new in the U.S.; many of the therapists educated prior to the 1990s will not have studied the vestibular system, exercises for vestibular disorders, or canalith repositioning unless they took continuing education courses after graduation. Many physical therapists may know little or nothing about vestibular rehabilitation or treatments to specifically stop BPPV. Insurance requirements, economic concerns, or other factors may result in your being sent to a therapist with limited vestibular knowledge or experience.

If you are sent to a physical therapist, you can ask how long she or he has worked with people with vestibular problems and how many such people he or she has seen. You might ask if the therapist has seen anyone in a situation like yours before or has treated BPPV.

Occupational Therapist

According to the Occupational Therapy Association, occupational therapists help people restore and sustain a productive life after setbacks from illness or injury. They also help people cope with developmental disabilities or with changes related to aging.

These therapists use "occupation" or "purposeful activity" as a means of preventing, reducing, or overcoming physical, social, and emotional disabilities in people of all ages.

To become an occupational therapist, one must have a bachelor's degree or master's degree in occupational therapy. To practice in most jobs and most states, occupational therapists must pass a nationally administered test and be licensed. After that, they can use the title of occupational therapist, registered (OTR).

Not all occupational therapists have had education, training, or experience in vestibular disorders. If you are sent for an occupational therapy assessment, you can ask how long the therapist has worked with people with vestibular problems, how many people she or he has worked with, and if the therapist has worked with anyone in a situation like yours before.

Registered Nurse

A registered nurse (RN) has completed the nursing program at a state-accredited junior college or university, passed a nationally administered examination, and is licensed to practice nursing by a state board of nursing.

Registered nurses can be considered generalists who know a little bit about many aspects of health care. They can record your history, assess your current condition, administer medication, take blood, start an IV, change bandages, remove stitches, and teach/inform you about your testing and diagnosis and about treatments such as diet, drugs, and stress reduction.

RNs generally have limited knowledge of the inner ear and its functions unless they have had extra training and education in this area.

Others at the Doctor's Office

Not everyone working for the doctor is a nurse. Doctors may use trained employees, medical assistants, licensed practical nurses (LPNs), or registered nurses to complete medical office tasks independently or in a doctor's presence.

Mental Health Professionals

Some people with BPPV feel an acute loss of control and, possibly, depression. Seeing a psychiatrist or psychologist may be recommended.

Psychiatrist

A psychiatrist is an M.D. who specializes in psychiatry after completing a psychiatric residency training program. A psychiatrist usually does not have any specific training in BPPV or other vestibular disorders.

Psychologist

A psychologist is someone with college degrees in psychology. He or she will usually have a Ph.D. in some area of psychology and will have spent eight or more years studying psychology in college. It would be unusual if this professional had any training or experience in BPPV or any other vestibular disorder.

Summary

While dealing with BPPV, you may encounter many health care professionals. Don't assume they know anything about BPPV or the vestibular system. Ask if they have been trained in this area and if they are seeing other patients with symptoms and problems like yours.

References

_____. *The Official ABMS Directory of Board Certified Medical Specialists, Vol. 3: Otolaryngologists*. 28th edition. Illinois: Marquis, 1995.

American Neurotology Society, "The American Neurotology Society," http://itsa.ucsf.edu/~ajo/ANS/Policies/Policy.html. June 6, 1997.

American Occupational Therapy Association (AOTA), "Member Information," http://www.aota.org/membinfo.html. June 6, 1997.

American Academy of Otolaryngology-Head and Neck Surgery. "What Is an Otolaryngologist-Head and Neck Surgeon?" (public service brochure), 1994.

American Speech-Language-Hearing Association (ASHA), *Membership and Certification Handbook-Audiology*, 1994.

Cohen, H., Rubin, A.M., and Gombash, L. "The Team Approach to Treatment of the Dizzy Patient." *Archives of Physical Medicine and Rehabilitation*, 73:703-708, 1992.

Naifeh, S., and Smith, G.W. *The Best Doctors in America*. South Carolina: Woodward/White, 1994.

Wolfe, S., Gabay, M., McCarthy, P., Bame, A., and Adler, B.M. *Questionable Doctors: A Public Citizen Health Research Group Report*, March 1996.

Chapter 14

Insurance

If you have BPPV, you will find it useful to know something about health insurance coverage offered by traditional insurers, Health Maintenance Organizations (HMOs), Preferred Provider Organizations (PPOs), the Consolidated Omnibus Budget Reconciliation Act of 1985 (COBRA), Medicare, and Medicaid. You may also want to know about disability insurance, including Social Security Disability Insurance.

Note: This chapter will be relevant mainly to people living in the U.S. Health insurance plans in other countries vary greatly, and explaining them lies beyond the scope of this book.

Health Insurance

Health insurance comes in many varieties and with a staggering number of rules and regulations. It can be divided generally into traditional insurance coverage, PPOs, HMOs, Medicaid, and Medicare. The information below will give you an overview of health insurance. Refer to your insurance policy for any specific information you may need about benefits, rules, and regulations.

PPO Health Insurance

Preferred provider organization (PPO) health insurance usually allows you to visit any doctor in any place, but your out-of-pocket expense will be lower if you choose someone on the PPO's list of preferred providers. The list generally includes doctors, hospitals, labs, radiology offices, and other health-care professionals and agencies.

A typical arrangement is for the PPO to pay 90 percent and for you to pay 10 percent of the bills for treatment by a preferred provider. If you choose a non-preferred provider for treatment, the PPO will pay less, and you will pay more.

HMO Health Insurance

Insurance from a health maintenance organization (HMO)

involves a membership contract between you and the organization. By joining, you are allowing the HMO to decide what health care you will receive and from whom. If you want the HMO to pay for your medical bills, your choice is limited to those providers, facilities, and hospitals under contract with that particular HMO. Your bills will not be paid if you seek care outside of the HMO while you are living at home. Different rules apply when you are traveling.

Some HMOs hire their own doctors and specialists and buy or create their own clinics and hospitals. Other HMOs may hire MDs and make contracts with hospitals and other health-care agencies that are independent of the HMO.

Most HMOs have stringent rules about using emergency room services. They do not want to pay emergency room rates for non-emergency problems. For example, here is one insurance company's list of health conditions or situations that constitute an emergency:

- uncontrolled bleeding
- severe burns
- seizure or loss of consciousness
- broken bones
- severe shortness of breath
- inability to swallow
- suspected drug overdose or poisoning
- chest pain or severe squeezing sensation in the chest
- stroke symptoms such as sudden paralysis, suddenly slurred speech, numbness or paralysis of arm or leg, lack of responsiveness, severe headache

If you have BPPV and belong to an HMO, you should ask your doctor ahead of time if and when you should go to the emergency room for the symptoms of BPPV. Sometimes HMOs have refused to pay emergency room bills for problems they did not define as emergencies.

Traditional Health Insurance

With traditional health insurance, you pay a monthly premium, and the insurance company pays a percentage of your medical bills. The percentage the insurance company pays is determined by the individual policy. Usually, you are responsible for the first $250 to $500 of charges (the deductible) each year. After the deductible limit is reached, the insurer will usually pay 80 percent of a "reasonable and customary" charge as defined by the insurance company, and you will pay 20 percent. With this kind of policy, the insurer places no restrictions on which doctor you see. Generally, this type of health insurance is the most expensive, and it is the least likely to be available from your employer.

Medicare

Medicare is a kind of U.S. Federal health insurance available to people receiving Social Security retirement benefits or Social Security disability benefits.

People are automatically eligible for Medicare after receiving Social Security disability benefits for two years. Enrollment in Medicare decreases the monthly disability check by the relatively small cost of the Medicare premium.

Medicare coverage includes various options, including using an HMO. Get and read current Medicare publications before making any decisions about health insurance coverage. Keep in mind that if you don't enroll for Medicare when it is first offered to you, you will pay a much higher premium if you enroll later.

Medicaid

Medicaid is a kind of governmental health insurance for the indigent. Both the U.S. Federal government and individual state governments fund this insurance. Because of this setup, Medicaid eligibility and benefits can differ significantly from state to state.

Generally, to qualify for Medicaid your monthly income must be very low and your bank accounts must be very small.

Common Health Insurance Terms

Authorization, pre-authorization, or *referral* are terms used by insurers to mean the process of granting official permission to see a specialist or have a test or procedure done that can't be done by your primary care doctor. This permission may be given verbally or in writing. Different health plans have different rules; ask about them when you are told to go for specialty care or testing. It's always best to get this permission in writing and to double-check its validity with the insurance company.

Pre-certification is another term used to mean the process of getting official permission from your insurance company for something such as an MRI (or other equally expensive test) or surgery. Pre-certification has become routine with most insurers, including Medicare, Medicaid, PPOs, and traditional health insurers.

A *co-payment* or *co-insurance* refers to a fixed amount of money you pay for a visit to the doctor's office, usually $5 to $10, in addition to the money paid for the visit by your insurance.

A *deductible* is the total amount of money you must spend on your annual health care bills before your insurance company begins to pay. Only health care covered by your insurance policy counts toward the total.

In-patient and *out-patient* are important terms because some insurance companies pay at one rate for out-patient tests and procedures and at another rate for in-patient. These two terms have blurred significantly over the last several years. Staying overnight in the hospital used to define the difference; now you may be considered an out-patient even if your hospital stay is as much as 23 hours and includes one night.

Medically necessary is a term used to describe whether or not your insurance company considers a test, office visit, procedure, or treatment necessary given your diagnosis and condition. Whether or not your primary doctor or specialist thinks it is needed is not the question.

Insurers use *usual and customary, usual and prevailing,* or *allowable* to mean what, in their view, something should cost. This is not necessarily what your doctor charges or what anyone else has charged you.

Privacy

Insurance companies almost always insist upon having full access to your medical records as a pre-requisite to paying your claim. In many cases, you will be asked to sign a form giving your doctor permission to send any requested part of your medical record to your insurance company. The only way you can avoid this loss of privacy is to pay for your own care.

COBRA

If you are unable to perform your job and leave work of your own accord or you are fired, you may be eligible to maintain your employee health insurance policy through the Consolidated Omnibus Budget Reconciliation Act of 1985 (COBRA). This Federal law requires any employer with 20 or more employees to offer continued health insurance after an employee has left a job. The coverage must usually be provided for 18 months, possibly more under certain circumstances. This act does not require the employer to pay for the coverage, only to provide the departing employee with the opportunity to buy it. In order to qualify, you must sign up within 60 days of leaving your job.

Disability Insurance

Only an extremely small number of people with a diagnosis of BPPV will become disabled to the point of being unable to continue working for pay. According to the 1995 annual report of the National

Institute on Deafness and Other Communication Disorders, during 1994 only an estimated 7,600 people throughout the U.S. received Social Security benefits (Social Security Disability Insurance payments and Supplemental Security Income payments combined) for balance problems, including those caused by BPPV. These were the most recent figures available in late 1999.

Note about working: Try to continue working if you can, safely. Usually, Social Security disability payments and private disability insurance will not come close to matching your normal paycheck. Also, even if you qualify for Social Security disability, you will not be eligible for health insurance from Medicare until two years later.

Disability benefits may be available from a private insurance policy and/or the government via the Social Security Administration for people unable to keep their jobs.

Benefits from private policies differ from situation to situation. Most policies have a choice of elimination periods (the varying periods of time that must go by before certain benefits begin) and different amounts of payment. These policies are usually set up to cover you for a short time until you qualify for Social Security disability benefits.

If you did not buy a private disability insurance policy on your own, check to see if you have such coverage through your employer. (Sometimes such coverage is referred to as "short term disability.")

Social Security

Note: This section of the book contains quotes, not the entire texts, from Social Security publications. You should obtain and read current Social Security publications in their entirety before applying for or making decisions about Social Security. See "For More Information" later in this chapter for Social Security's central phone numbers and its World Wide Web address, or visit your local branch.

Disability Definition

According to the Social Security Administration, "Disability under Social Security is based on your inability to work. You will be considered disabled if you are unable to do any kind of work for which you are suited and your disability is expected to last for at least a year or to result in death."

Social Security Programs

The Social Security Administration oversees two different programs related to disability, Social Security Disability Insurance (SSDI) and Supplemental Security Income (SSI). The same process for each program determines a person's disability, but the financial eligibility differs. Financial eligibility for SSDI payments is based on how much you have contributed to Social Security over time. On the other hand, SSI payments are made on the basis of your current financial need, and your past contributions to Social Security are not taken into account. Social Security Publication No. 05-11000 has more information.

These two Social Security programs are set up to begin six months after the start of the kind of disability defined above. It is assumed that people will have their own contingency plans to support them during a disability of less than one year.

Although the disability must go on for at least a year to qualify, your benefits could begin to accumulate before the one-year date. For example, suppose that in January 1998 you became unable to work. In June 1998, you applied for Social Security benefits. A year later, in June 1999, benefits are approved. In this case, you will be paid retroactively (in a lump sum) for each month between June 1998 and June 1999, and you will also begin to receive ongoing monthly benefits. If your initial application were rejected, *and* you chose to appeal, *and* you used a lawyer during the appeal stage, *and* you won your appeal, a predetermined percentage of this lump sum would go for the lawyer's services.

When to Apply

There is no general answer to the question of when to apply for Social Security disability benefits. A diagnosis of BPPV or any type of vestibular disorder does not automatically make you eligible for a disability benefit; you must also meet the Social Security Administration's definition of "disabled." Someone who fits the definition and has been unable to work for five months or more would have the greatest chance of obtaining disability benefits.

How to Apply

You can apply at a Social Security office by phone or mail. According to a Social Security publication, "Social Security disability benefits will not begin until the sixth full month of disability. This waiting period begins with the first full month after the date we decide your disability began." The application process will usually require 60 to 90 days.

Application Requirements

For the application process, you need all of the following:

• names, addresses, and phone numbers of doctors, hospitals, clinics, and institutions that treated you; dates of treatment

• names of all the medications you are taking

• medical records from your doctors, therapists, hospitals, clinics, and caseworkers, including laboratory and test results

• a summary of where you worked in the past 15 years and the kind of work you did

• a copy of your W-2 Form (Wage and Tax Statement), or if you are self-employed, your Federal tax return for the past year

The Review Process

According to a Social Security publication called "Social Security Disability Benefits," the Social Security office will review your application:

> "to see if you are eligible to apply for disability benefits. These include such factors as whether you have worked long enough and recently enough to qualify for disability benefits, your age, and, if you are applying for benefits as a family member, your relationship to the worker. The office will then send your application to the Disability Determination Services (DDS) office in your state. There, a decision will be made as to whether you are disabled under the Social Security law.
>
> "In the DDS office, a team consisting of a physician (or psychologist) and a disability evaluation specialist will consider all the facts in your case and decide if you are disabled. They will use the medical evidence from your doctors and from hospitals, clinics, or institutions where you have been treated.
>
> "On the medical report forms, your doctors or other sources are asked for a medical history of your condition: what is wrong with you; when it began; how it limits your activities; what the medical tests have shown; and what treatment has been provided. They are also asked for information about your ability to do work-related activities, such as walking, sitting, lifting, and carrying. They are not asked to decide whether you are disabled.
>
> "Additional medical information may be needed before the DDS team can decide your case. If it is not available from

your current medical sources, you may be asked to take a special examination called a consultative examination. Your doctor or the medical facility where you have been treated is the preferred source to perform this examination. Social Security will pay for the examination or any other additional medical tests you may need, and for certain travel expenses related to it."

SSA officials use a Social Security publication entitled, "Disability Evaluation Under Social Security" to help determine disability.

The Appeals Process

According to another SSA publication, "The Appeals Process,"

"If your claim is denied or you disagree with any other decision we make, you may appeal the decision. The Social Security office will help you complete the paperwork.

"There are four levels of appeal. If you disagree with the decision at one level, you may appeal to the next level. You have 60 days from the time you receive the decision to file an appeal to the next level. We assume that you receive the decision five days after the date on it, unless you can show us that you received it later. For more information about appeals, ask for the fact sheet, (Publication No. 05-10041)."

Hiring a Lawyer

Whether to hire a lawyer or not is a choice you must make for yourself. Keep in mind that you can't use a lawyer unless you have been turned down by Social Security and have decided to appeal. If you use a lawyer, you will probably be asked to give him or her a percentage of the money you may be owed by the Social Security Administration.

For More Information

According to Social Security,

"You can get more information 24 hours a day by calling Social Security's toll-free number: 1-800-772-1213. You can speak to a service representative between the hours of 7 a.m. and 7 p.m. on business days. Pre-recorded information and services also are available during and after normal business hours.

"If you want to speak to a representative, it's best to call later in the week and later in the month. When you call, have your Social Security number handy.

"Hearing-impaired callers using TTY equipment can reach Social Security between 7 a.m. and 7 p.m. weekdays by calling 1-800-325-0778."

Here are some booklets you can obtain from the Social Security Administration:

- "SSI" (Publication No. 05-11000) explains the Supplemental Security Income program, which provides a basic income to people who are 65 or older, disabled, or blind, and have limited income and resources.
- "Benefits for Children with Disabilities" (Publication No. 05-10026) explains benefits available to children with disabilities.
- "Working While Disabled . . . How We Can Help" (Publication No. 05-10095)-explains work incentives for Social Security and SSI beneficiaries.

Social Security information is also available to users of the Internet. To view Social Security information on the World Wide Web of the Internet, go to http://www.ssa.gov.

Avoiding Problems

You can do the following things to avoid problem with your application:

- Tell your doctor what is happening to you. You are the only one who knows how you feel and how your functioning has been affected. This must be communicated to your doctor. Keep a journal of your problems and how many days you are taking off from work. No test will show your disability; you must report it to your doctor. Do not assume someone knows what you are going through; BPPV and associated problems are different from case to case.
- Get a true advocate. Sometimes the medical record is a problem because your doctor doesn't believe you or thinks your symptoms are not as bad as you say. If this becomes the case, you need to look for someone more experienced in dealing with inner ear problems who can act as an advocate.
- Seek follow-up care. An on-going medical record is needed to retain Social Security disability benefits. To maintain such a record, you must see a doctor at somewhat regular intervals.

References

______. Public Health Service, U.S. Department of Health and Human Services, National Institutes of Health, *Research in Human Communication: 1995 Annual Report of the National Institute on Deafness and Other Communication Disorders*. NIDCD:Bethesda, Md., 1997.

______. Social Security Administration, U.S. Department of Health and Human Services. "Social Security Disability Benefits." SSA Publication No. 05-10029, May 1996.

______. Social Security Administration, U.S. Department of Health and Human Services. "Disability Evaluation Under Social Security." SSA Publication No. 64-039, Jan. 1995.

Delk, J.H. *Comprehensive Dictionary of Audiology*. Sioux City Iowa: The Hearing Aid Journal, 1973.

Chapter 15
Research

Because not everything about BPPV is known, research is still needed. Many people carry out research in the U.S. and worldwide. Ph.D.s, M.D.s, physical therapists, occupational therapists, and others conduct research in universities, hospitals, institutes, and doctors' offices. Research money comes from varied sources.

Few studies have targeted BPPV alone. However, studies of other vestibular problems and other medical disciplines have sometimes provided useful information.

Who Is in Charge?

"Nobody" is the short answer to the question of who's in charge of BPPV research. There is no central person or organization issuing general orders. However, those handling the research money have a great deal of influence over what is studied.

Organizations such as the U.S. Federal government or the Deafness Research Foundation (DRF), which fund research by competition for grants, generally have long-term goals or objectives formulated by groups of research scientists. Researchers, guided by the goals and findings of previous research, devise projects and try to write compelling research proposals. Funding organizations usually choose projects on the basis of how well they will help meet organization goals, how they are designed, and which have the best chance of collecting valuable data.

Scientists are said to compete for funds, and this is accurate. The winners of this competition get the research money, and the others do not.

Funding Sources

Both private and public sources provide funds for study of BPPV and other vestibular disorders.

Non-governmental sources of funds include nonprofit organizations like the DRF, the American Otological Society, and the National Organization for Hearing Research. Corporations such as medical equipment companies also sometimes support research related to their products.

Federal Government

The Federal government, via the National Institutes of Health (NIH), is the largest source of funds for vestibular research in the U.S. Other agencies such as the National Science Foundation (NSF), the National Aeronautics and Space Administration (NASA), the Veteran's Administration, and the U.S. Navy also fund projects dealing with vestibular disorders and balance in general.

NIH

The NIH, headquartered in Bethesda, Maryland, is the largest Federal agency for biomedical research. In 1996, the total budget for research activities by the NIH was $12 billion (for all research activities, not for vestibular disorders). Congress sets the total budget for the NIH and other Federal agencies.

The NIH is one of eight agencies of the Public Health Service within the U.S. Department of Health and Human Services.

The mission of the NIH is "to uncover new knowledge that will lead to better health for everyone." It carries out this mission by awarding money for research projects, by financing science training, by providing funds for beginning researchers, and by funding centers for training in research. Only a small amount of this work is conducted at its Maryland home; the rest is done in locations throughout the country.

The NIH is divided into 18 different institutes including the National Institute on Deafness and Other Communication Disorders (NIDCD). The other institutes deal with cancer, vision, genome studies, aging, dental studies, heart/lung/blood studies, alcohol abuse/alcoholism, allergies/infectious diseases, arthritis/musculoskeletal/skin diseases, child health/human development, drug abuse, diabetes/digestion/kidneys, environmental health sciences, general medical sciences, mental health, neurological disorders/stroke, and nursing research.

NIDCD

The NIH institute overseeing inner ear research is the National Institute on Deafness and Other Communication Disorders (NIDCD), headed by James. F. Battey, Jr., M.D., Ph.D. The NIDCD's areas of responsibility include research on hearing, balance, smell, taste, language, voice, and speech.

During fiscal year 1994, 4 percent of the NIDCD budget went for vestibular studies and 57 percent for hearing. During fiscal year 1995, 7 percent ($9.1 million) of the NIDCD budget went for the study of balance and 53 percent for hearing. (The other funding included 10 percent for smell, 5 percent for taste, 5 percent for voice, 9 percent for speech, and 11 percent for language.) The fiscal year 1997 appropriation (budget amount) from Congress was for $188 million, a 6.8 percent ($12 million) increase over fiscal year 1996.

Because vestibular function is so important and because vestibular disturbances can cause problems in many areas of the body, other institutes also fund research related to balance. In 1995, the National Eye Institute spent $4.7 million, NASA $4.4 million, and the National Institute on Aging $2.5 million. These were funds spent on balance research in general.

NIDCD goals for balance are developed and published as the National Strategic Research Plan for balance every six years. This plan describes progress in balance research and outlines areas of need. The most recent plan was written for 1994-1995. Areas identified for further study included the following:

- ion transport
- neurotransmitters
- normal development
- aging
- hair cell regeneration
- genetics
- gaze control
- posture control
- spatial orientation
- diagnostic testing
- immune reactions/diseases
- autonomic nervous system control
- physical therapy
- aminoglycoside destruction procedures
- monitoring during inner ear surgeries
- a better animal model to study
- fluid transport in epithelial tissues other than the ear

To partially fulfill its goals, the NIDCD funds six large ongoing projects, as follows:

- national multipurpose research and training center for balance at the University of California at Los Angeles (UCLA)
- national multipurpose research and training center for hearing and balance at Johns Hopkins University
- national research and training center for childhood deafness at the Boys Town National Research Hospital
- NIDCD Information Clearinghouse for the dispersal of information to the public
- National Temporal Bone, Hearing and Balance Pathology Resource Registry to promote temporal bone donation and research

- NIDCD/NASA multi-institutional center for vestibular research at the Robert S. Dow Neurological Sciences Institute in Portland and Northwestern University in Chicago.

Applied Research

Research is a long process that may or may not lead to practical applications. Findings may be applied by some doctors and not by others. No central authority coordinates the application of research results.

A great deal of time and effort go into competing for grants and grant renewals. The research may take years to complete. Presenting studies and findings at professional meetings and in medical journals, scientific journals, and books takes still more time. Eventually the new information may be available to help solve particular practical problems. Each physician providing medical care determines what new research findings might be useful in his or her practice. What gets used is highly individual and depends upon many factors including the doctor' s clinical experience and what he or she learned in medical school and during residency and fellowship training. Other factors would include what the doctor thinks about research, the meeting or book or journal presenting the research, and requests made by particular patients.

How to Encourage Research

Here are ways to encourage BPPV research:

- In the U.S., help keep NIH funding at present levels or above by writing to your U.S. Representative and U.S. Senators and to the Senate and House appropriations committees.
- In the U.S., help keep National Science Foundation funding at present levels or above by writing to your U.S. Representative and U.S. Senators.
- In the U.S., sign up with the Temporal Bone Registry to donate your own temporal bones to science for possible study after you die. (See "Temporal Bone Research and Donation" later in this chapter.)
- Give money to organizations that fund research. (See Chapter 16, "Where to Get More Information.")

Research Projects

Few research studies are looking specifically at BPPV, but a large number are investigating the vestibular system in general. Some of these may discover things about BPPV.

NIH-Funded Projects

Current NIH funded research includes:

- *Treatments for Benign Paroxysmal Positional Vertigo* -- Helen Cohen, OTR, Ph.D., Baylor University, Houston, Tex.; human research funded from 1998 through July 2003.

The aim of this research is to:

1. Compare the canalith repositioning maneuver (CRP), the Semont maneuver, and Brandt-Daroff exercises to each other and to a sham treatment.
2. Compare habituation exercises with CRP, the Semont maneuver, Brandt-Daroff exercises, and with a sham treatment.
3. Determine if variations of the above treatments lessen or improve their effectiveness.
4. Determine the effect of additional conditions on short- and long-term response to treatment.

Information like this should help health care professionals determine the best BPPV treatment for an individual.

- *Imaging the Cupula and Semicircular Canal in Situ* -- Robert Silver, Washington University, St Louis, Mo.; toadfish research funded from 1994 through 2004. This research may improve understanding of how the cupula works, and this could lead to improved diagnosis and treatment of BPPV.
- *Mechanics of Motion Transduction by the Semicircular Canals in the Toadfish*, Richard Rabbitt, Washington University, St Louis, Mo.; toadfish research funded from 1994 through 2004. The overall goal of this project is "to develop a mathematical model to determine the dynamics of the semicircular canal cupula and endolymph in the toadfish." A more complete understanding of endolymph and cupula movement may lead to a better understanding of what causes BPPV and how to treat it.

Recent Publications about Research

- "Efficacy of Treatments for Posterior Canal Benign Paroxysmal Positional Vertigo," Helen S. Cohen, Ph.D., OTR, and Jaroslav Jerabek, *Laryngoscope*, 109(4):584-90, 1999. This study by researchers from Baylor University in Houston, Tex., and Charles University in Prague, Czech Republic, compared three treatments for BPPV: modified CRP, modified CRP with augmented head movements, and modified Semont maneuver.
- "Postural Control in Benign Paroxysmal Positional Vertigo Before and After Recovery," Stefano Di Girolamo, *et al.*, *Acta Otolaryngologica (Stockh)*, 118(3):289-293, 1998. A research team at Catholic University of Rome, Italy, performed computerized

dynamic posturography on people with BPPV before and after they were treated with the Semont maneuver.

- "Benign Positioning Vertigo (BPV) and Three-Dimensional (3-D) Eye Movement Analysis," G. Dumas, R. Charachon, and J.P. Lavielle, *Acta Oto-Rhino-Laryngologica, Belg.*, 52:291-307, 1998. Scientists at Centre Hospitalier Albert Michallon in Grenoble, France, studied the use of computer analyzed infrared photography in cases of BPPV.
- "Recognition and Management of Horizontal Canal Benign Positional Vertigo," Terry Fife, M.D., *American Journal of Otology,* 19(3):345-351, 1998. Dr. Fife conducted his study at Barrow Neurological Institute in Phoenix, Ariz.
- "Treatment of Benign Positional Vertigo Using Heels-Over-Head Rotation," Furman, J.M., Cass, S.P., and Briggs, B.C., *Annals of Otology, Rhinology and Laryngology*, 107:1046-1053, 1999. The authors, based at the University of Pittsburgh, Pennsylvania, looked at an experimental treatment method that limits neck movement during CRP.
- "Epley's Manoeuvre for Benign Paroxysmal Positional Vertigo: A Prospective Study," M. Wolf, et al., *Clinical Otolaryngology*, 24:43-46, 1999. The researchers conducted this study at Tel Aviv University in Israel.

Research Presented at Professional Meetings

American Otological Society - 1998

- *Paroxysmal Positional Vertigo Syndrome*. Vicente Honrubia, M.D., D.M.Sc., Marjorie R. Harris, M.A., and Robert W. Baloh, M.D., of the University of California Los Angeles (U.C.L.A.) investigated the differential diagnosis of patients with benign paroxysmal positional vertigo (BPPV) originating in various canals by testing with infrared video cameras after Hallpike tests. Their conclusion was that, "the location of the BPPV pathology can be diagnosed on the basis of nystagmus reactions to Hallpike tests directed to specific semicircular canals."
- "Paroxysmal Positional Vertigo: Idiopathic vs. Post-Traumatic," Athanasios Katsarkas, M.D., M.Sc., of McGill University, Quebec, Canada, looked at the cases of BPPV treated at his clinic. He found that 15.5 percent of the patients visiting his dizziness clinic had BPPV. Diagnosis was established by clinical examination; posterior canal BPPV was most common; the post-traumatic BPPV group differed from the idiopathic group in age, ratio of women to men, and unilateral to bilateral occurrence.

- "Treatment of Peripheral and Central Positional Vertigo Utilizing Repositioning, Redistribution, and Habituation Techniques," Ronald L. Steenerson, M.D., and Gaye W. Cronin, MHE, OTR, Atlanta, Ga.
- "Mastoid Oscillation in Canalith Repositioning for Paroxysmal Positional Vertigo," John W. Currens, M.D.; Aukse E. Bankaitis, Ph.D., and Eric W. Sargent, M.D.
- "Prevalence of Benign Paroxysmal Positional Vertigo in Meniere's Disease," Gerard J. Gianoli, M.D, and Brooks Brennan, B.S., Tulane University, La.
- "Vestibular Testing in Benign Paroxysmal Positional Vertigo," Darin V. Sutton, M.D.; Barry Strasnick, M.D.; John Jacobson, Ph.D., Norfolk, Va. Follow-up caloric testing was done in people who tested abnormal before treatment with CRP. Of the eight who were retested after CRP, four returned to normal.

Association for Research in Otolaryngology, 1999

- "Effects of Exercise on Prevention of Recurrence of BPPV Symptoms," M. Amin, Marian Girardi, M. Neill, L.F. Hughes, and Horst Konrad, M.D., Southern Illinois University, Springfield, Ill. The researchers examined two groups of people who had had successful CRP treatment. One group did nothing special after the CRP, and one performed Brandt-Daroff exercises. Those performing the exercises became much less symptomatic than those not performing them.

Temporal Bone Research and Donation

The temporal bone is a part of the skull that houses the outer, middle, and inner ears. One of the best ways to study the inner ear is to examine the temporal bone after death. Such bones are obtained from people who have donated or pledged their temporal bones for research after their death. A small part of the temporal bone (only the part containing the middle and inner ears) is surgically removed soon after death. This removal does not affect the appearance of the donor's outer ear, face, or head. The temporal bone is then prepared for a variety of research techniques.

The standard technique consists of light microscopy, which involves the following steps: fixing the temporal bone in formalin to preserve the various delicate structures of the inner ear, decalcifying the bone to soften it, infiltrating the bone with a substance like celloidin so that it can be sectioned, sectioning or slicing the bone, and finally, staining it with haematoxylin and eosin. Each temporal bone usually yields 400 to 500 serial sections, of which about 40 are selected and stained for study. The other non-stained sections are saved for future use. This technique of preparation for light microscopy needs special equipment and expertise, is time consuming, tedious, and expensive. For example, it takes approximately two years and $1,000 to $2,000 per bone. However, such study is well worth the time and the expense because it can yield a tremendous amount of useful information that cannot be obtained in any other way. There are only a handful of laboratories in the United States and in the world which perform such temporal bone research.

Besides standard light microscopy and surface preparations, a variety of newer research techniques such as DNA studies have been developed in the past several years that have enhanced the value of this type of research. These newer techniques include electron microscopy, immuno-staining, computer-aided reconstruction, and procedures that allow identification of defects at a molecular level (molecular biology). The newer techniques hold promise in providing clues and answers to many of the mysteries of BPPV and other disorders affecting the inner ear.

Donating Your Temporal Bones

Persons affected by BPPV can contribute to advances in understanding and treating it by pledging to donate their temporal bones for research purposes after death. Such research will make it possible to provide others with the gift of balance and hearing in the future. People who wish to donate their temporal bones can do so by contacting the NIDCD National Temporal Bone Registry and enrolling in its National Temporal Bone Donor Program. Those who donate their temporal bones should also consider donating the brain stem, where some of the brain pathways for balance and hearing are located.

National Temporal Bone Registry

The NIDCD National Temporal Bone, Hearing and Balance Pathology Resource Registry is a nonprofit organization. It was established in 1992 by the National Institute on Deafness and Other Communication Disorders (NIDCD) of the National Institutes of Health, the Federal government's focal point for biomedical and behavioral research on hearing and balance. The Registry continues and expands on the activities of the former National Temporal Bone Banks Program, which was created in 1960 to encourage temporal bone donation. The Registry serves both the public and the scientific community by providing the following resources and services:

- enrollment of temporal bone donors
- 24-hour nationwide network to collect temporal bones after a donor's death
- computerized database of all human temporal bone collections in the United States
- dissemination of public information on temporal bone donation
- publication of a semi-annual newsletter, *The Registry*
- conservation of existing human temporal bone collections
- professional educational activities to teach physicians and scientists about temporal bone research

The Registry's national office is located at the Massachusetts Eye and Ear Infirmary in Boston. The Registry works closely with all of the nation's 26 temporal bone research laboratories listed below:

Armed Forces Institute of Pathology/Walter Reed Army Medical Center, Washington, D.C.
Baylor College of Medicine, Houston, Texas
Bowman Gray School of Medicine, Winston-Salem, North Carolina
Columbia-Presbyterian Medical Center, New York, New York
Goodhill Ear Center-UCLA School of Medicine, Los Angeles, California
Henry Ford Hospital, Detroit, Michigan
House Ear Institute, Los Angeles, California
J. Hillis Miller Health Center, Gainesville, Florida
Kresge Hearing Research Institute-University of Michigan, Ann Arbor, Michigan
Massachusetts Eye and Ear Infirmary, Boston, Massachusetts
Mt. Sinai School of Medicine, New York, New York
New England Medical Center Hospitals, Boston, Massachusetts
New York University, New York, New York
Northwestern University Medical School, Chicago, Illinois
Otological Research Laboratories, Columbus, Ohio
Shea Clinic Foundation, Memphis, Tennessee
SUNY Health Science Center, Syracuse, New York
The Eye and Ear Institute of Pittsburgh, Pittsburgh, Pennsylvania
The Johns Hopkins University, Baltimore, Maryland
The University of Iowa Hospitals and Clinics, Iowa City, Iowa
University of Chicago, Chicago, Illinois
University of Colorado Health Science Center, Denver, Colorado
University of Minnesota, Minneapolis, Minnesota
University of Oklahoma Health Sciences Center, Oklahoma City, Oklahoma
University of Texas Southwestern Medical Center, Dallas, Texas
University of Wisconsin Hospital, Madison, Wisconsin

Questions about Donation

Here are common questions and their answers regarding temporal bone donations. If you have other questions, please contact the Temporal Bone Registry for further information.

Is there an age restriction?

No. No one is too young or too old to be a donor. Age does not affect the scientific value of your temporal bones.

Does removal of the temporal bones change the donor's appearance?

No. Removal of the temporal bones (and brain stem) does not change the appearance of the head, face, or outer ear. So, it does not affect funeral or burial arrangements, including an open casket.

Is there a cost to the donor's family or estate?

No. The medical professionals who remove the temporal bones donate their time or are paid by the laboratory receiving the temporal bones.

Is an autopsy necessary?

The consent form in your temporal bone donor packet gives permission for a limited autopsy for temporal bone (and related brain tissue) removal. In special circumstances, temporal bones may be removed without an autopsy.

Can I donate my body to science for anatomical study and also donate my temporal bones?

It depends. The policies of donor programs for anatomical study vary. Discuss this with your local body donor program to determine whether it is possible to donate to one or both programs.

Can I donate other organs for transplantation as well as my temporal bones?

Yes. The removal of your temporal bones would simply be delayed a few hours so that transplantable organs can be removed first.

What is the role of my next of kin?

In most states, the next of kin makes the final decision about organ or body donations. Inform them and your doctors of your wish to be a temporal bone donor. Be sure that they understand that their cooperation is needed.

How to Enroll as a Donor

- Contact the Registry by calling its 24-hour toll-free number (800) 822-1327 (voice) or (617) 573-3888 (TTY) or by e-mail at tbregistry@meei.harvard.edu. The Registry will send you a donor enrollment packet, which includes a medical history questionnaire and a donation and consent form.
- Return the completed forms, and the Registry will send you a wallet-size Donor Card that states you are a temporal bone donor. The card also states that at the time of your death, your doctor or next of kin should call the Registry day or night at (800) 822-1327. The Registry will then coordinate the removal of your temporal bones.
- The Registry keeps a computerized record of all donations. It will also forward a copy of your pledge to the collaborating laboratory that is located nearest to you. This laboratory will eventually receive your temporal bones for study.
- Tell your family and doctors about your plans to donate. Your next of kin makes the final decision about donation, so make certain family members know of your wish to donate your temporal bones. Please be sure they understand that their cooperation is needed at the time of your death.
- Please keep the Registry informed of any change of address or change in your next of kin.
- Provide up-to-date medical records: The scientific value of your temporal bone donation is greatly enhanced if up-to-date medical records accompany it. Therefore, donors are encouraged to send records of all hearing tests, balance tests, and ear surgery to the Registry. Results of hearing tests (audiograms) that you may have had are extremely valuable. Researchers need your medical records so that they can correlate and link your symptoms to the changes they observe in your donated temporal bones.

References

______. *Annual Report-1995*. Bethesda, Md.: National Institute on Deafness and Other Communication Disorders (NIDCD).

______. *National Strategic Research Plan, 1994-1995: Language and Language Impairments, Balance and Balance Disorders, Voice and Voice Disorders* (NIH Publication No. 96-3217). Bethesda, Md.: National Institute on Deafness and Other Communication Disorders (NIDCD).

National Institutes of Health. "Notice Concerning the CRISP System on Gopher," http://www.nih.gov/grants/award/gophercrisp.htm. July 15, 1997.

Snow, J.B. "News from the National Institute on Deafness and Other Communication Disorders." *American Journal of Otology*, 15(2):132-136, 1996.

Snow, J.B. "News from the National Institute on Deafness and Other Communication Disorders." *American Journal of Otology*, 18(3): 285-287, 1997.

Chapter 16

Where to Get More Information

Your first source of information about BPPV and its diagnosis, treatment, and effects should always be your doctor and members of his or her staff. Additional information can also be found through libraries and from patient support organizations, the Internet (whether or not you own a computer), and other people with similar problems.

Libraries

The library has always been a good place to go for information. This is true even in the age of the Internet. You can find information about BPPV at the local hospital library, college library, and the closest medical school library. Your local library probably won't have any information about BPPV on its shelves but might be of help anyway.

Start with the librarian at your local library. She or he can make suggestions to help get you started. If the local library does not have the information you are looking for, the reference librarian or another librarian may be able to get it. Most libraries borrow books they don't own from libraries that have them (interlibrary loan). They can also help with access to the Internet.

Hospitals sometimes maintain medical libraries for their doctors and staffs, and sometimes these libraries are available for public use. On occasion, a hospital will have a library or a library section devoted to public education. These hospital libraries usually have a modest selection of books and scientific journals. Be prepared to do your own looking since hospital librarians may not have much time to assist you; their primary mission is to serve the hospital staff.

The local junior college may also have useful books and journals, particularly if it has a health care program for registered nurses, respiratory therapists, physical therapy assistants, or other health care professionals. Many four-year colleges and universities also have books, magazines, and scientific journals related to health care.

Medical schools usually have well-stocked medical libraries, and borrowing privileges may be available to the public. The information at these libraries will most likely be meant for graduate physicians, medical students, and students of other professional schools (nursing, audiology, physical therapy, pharmacy, occupational therapy, dentistry) associated with the college. If you are interested in reading medical and other health care journals, go prepared to make copies; journals usually can't be checked out of the library but must be used on the premises. Although medical school librarians may not have time to help you as much as public librarians, most of the medical libraries include displays and brochures explaining where things are and how to find them.

Some private clinics also make vestibular materials available to the public. For example, if you live near Los Angeles, you might find what you are looking for in the otology library at the House Ear Institute.

Organizations

A few organizations offer information to people about BPPV. Professional organizations, a patient support organization, research organizations, and the Federal government all distribute such information.

The Vestibular Disorders Association (VEDA) and the National Institute on Deafness and Other Communication Disorders (NIDCD) Information Clearinghouse are two good places to start. VEDA has a large collection of non-technical printed information as well as audiotapes and videotapes. It sends and receives e-mail and has a substantial Internet web site. It can also provide you with information about local support groups.

In the list below, lines containing the @ symbol are e-mail addresses. Lines beginning with http:// are addresses of sites on the World Wide Web of the Internet.

Patient Support Organizations

Brain Injury Association
1776 Mass. Ave. NW, #100; Washington, DC 20036
Phone: (202) 296-6443; Toll-Free: (800) 444-6443
76207.3114@compuserve.com

National Head Injury Foundation
1776 Massachusetts Ave. N.W. #100; Washington, D.C. 20036
(202) 296-6443; (800) 444-6443

National Mental Health Association
1021 Prince Street; Alexandria, VA 22314-2971
(703) 684-7722; Fax: (703) 684-7722
nmhainfo@aol.com; http://www.nmha.org

National Stroke Association
96 Inverness Dr. E., Ste. I; Englewood, CO 80112-5112
Phone: (303) 649-9299; Fax: (303) 649-1328
http://www.stroke.org/

Vestibular Disorders Association (VEDA)
P.O. Box 4467; Portland, OR 97208-4467
(503) 229-7705 (24-hour answering machine)
(800) 837-8428 (24-hour answering machine); Fax: (503) 229-8064
veda@vestibular.org; http://www.vestibular.org

Professional Organizations

American Academy of Neurology (AAN)
2221 University Ave. S.E., Ste. 335; Minneapolis, MN 55414
(800) 879-1960; (612) 623-8115; Fax: (612) 623-2491
aan@aan.com; http://www.aan.com

American Academy of Otolaryngology-Head and Neck Surgery
One Prince Street; Alexandria, VA 22314
Phone (703) 836-4444; TTY: (703) 519-1585; Fax: (703) 683-5100
entnews@aol.com; http://www.entnet.org/

American Physical Therapy Association
1111 N. Fairfax Street; Alexandria, VA 22314
Phone: (703) 684-2782, extension 8555; Toll-Free: (800) 999-2782
TTY: (703) 684-6748; Fax: (703) 684-7343
ablake@apta.org; http://www.apta.org/

American Psychiatric Association
Division of Public Affairs
1400 K Street, NW; Washington, DC 20005
Phone: (202) 682-6000
http://www.psych.org/index.html

American Psychological Association
750 First Street., NE; Washington, DC 20002-4242
Phone: (202) 336-5500; Toll-Free: (800) 374-2721
http://www.apa.org/

American-Speech-Language-Hearing Association (ASHA)
10801 Rockville Pike; Rockville, MD 20852-3279
Toll-Free: (800) 498-2071; Voice: (301) 897-5700
TTY: (301) 897-0157; Fax: (301) 571-0457
http://www.asha.org/

U. S. Government

National Library of Medicine
8600 Rockville Pike; Bethesda, MD 20894
Voice: (888) 346-3656
publicinfo@nlm.nih.gov; http://www.nlm.nih.gov/

NIDCD Information Clearinghouse
1 Communication Ave.; Bethesda, MD 20892-3456
Voice: (800) 241-1044; TDD/TT: (800) 241-1055;
Fax: (301) 907-8830
nidcdinfo@nidcd.nih.gov; http://www.nih.gov/nidcd/

NIDCD National Temporal Bone, Hearing, and Balance Pathology Resource Registry
Massachusetts Eye and Ear Infirmary
243 Charles St.; Boston, MA 02114-3096
Voice: (800) 822-1327; Voice: (617) 573-3711
TDD: (617) 573-3888; Fax: (617) 573-3838
tbregistry@meei.harvard.edu; http://www.tbregistry.org

Social Security Administration
(Check the telephone Yellow Pages for information on your local Social Security branch office.)
Voice: (800) 772-1213; TTY: (800) 325-0778
http://www.ssa.gov/reach.htm

Internet

If you have a computer and Internet access, you are probably already familiar with news groups, electronic mailing lists, web pages, and other electronic communication modes. Most of these modes can provide access to information about BPPV.

If you don't have a computer, try your local library. Most libraries have Internet access, and librarians can help you find things on the Internet.

If you don't have a computer, you can also ask neighbors and relatives who may have Internet access or know someone who does. Most people using the Internet would probably be happy to help you find information; part of their fun is the hunt.

Also, your town may have a "cyber cafe," a retail business offering Internet access in a coffeehouse setting.

Kinds of Information

The Internet includes an enormous amount of information. The U.S. Federal government has huge sites, including those of the Social Security Administration, the National Institute on Deafness and Other Communication Disorders (NIDCD), the National Institutes of Health (NIH), the National Library of Medicine (NLM), the Library of Congress and more. Information from many organizations, colleges and universities, hospitals, doctors, and individuals are available on the Internet. Many publishers of professional medical journals list the tables of contents of their journal issues; some even include summaries of the articles.

Government forms and publications are available "on-line" including booklets from the Social Security Administration. You can download them and print them immediately without writing a letter and waiting for a reply.

Books in print are listed at the Library of Congress Internet site, and medical books in print are listed at the NLM site.

A handful of universities have posted on-line textbooks containing basic anatomy and physiology of the ear and other ear information, including graphics, at their web sites.

If you want to read current scientific papers on BPPV and other topics, you can look for abstracts and bibliographic information on the Internet using MEDLINE, a database of the NLM. You can use the PubMed version on-line for free. MEDLINE contains more than 8.8 million references to articles published in 3,800 biomedical journals. Many of these references include 300-word abstracts as well as the names of titles, authors, publishers, and other bibliographic information. You can search MEDLINE at home or at work using your own computer and Internet connection, or you can use on-line services at libraries or other institutions offering web access to the public. To connect to PubMed or to find out more about it and other NLM services, go to the web page at http://www.nlm.nih.gov. Health care professionals and researchers as well as the general public use MEDLINE and related databases.

Other People with BPPV

How do you find other people with BPPV?

- First, ask at your doctor's office. Find out if the staff there can get permission for you to speak to another of their patients with BPPV. (If your ear specialist doesn't know of anyone else with similar problems, he or she isn't seeing many people with BPPV or other vestibular problems, and you might want to re-evaluate visiting this doctor).

- Ask your friends and relatives if they know of anyone with BPPV, and you might also try the clergy.
- If you are a VEDA member, you can ask other members for suggestions, stories, and advice via the VEDA pen pal lists, called Link Lists. VEDA's addresses are listed in the "Organizations" section earlier in this chapter.
- If you have Internet access, you can find others with similar problems through an electronic mailing list such as the Dizzinews mailing list

To join an electronic mailing list that includes people with BPPV, you must subscribe (for free) via e-mail. You must follow subscription directions exactly since a computer, not a person, handles the entire process. Unless you write the appropriate command in the correct place with the correct spelling, your e-mail subscription request will fail. If you are unsuccessful the first time, check your word placement and spelling. Delete all extraneous material, such as your automated signature lines, from your message. Here are examples:

Dizzinews Mailing List
To: majordomo@samurai.com
From: your e-mail address
Subject: (leave blank)
Message: subscribe dizzinews

Fill in the blanks as instructed and send the e-mail. The mailing list computer will send back a message to announce that you are subscribed and to tell you how the group works and how to quit the list (unsubscribe). Keep these instructions; save them on disk, and print a copy. You will need these instructions later if you want to unsubscribe.

Don't write anything to a group that you would not want on the front page of your local newspaper. Most e-mails sent to an entire group or mailing list are saved for anyone to read at any time.

Summary

When you need more information about some aspect of BPPV or its treatment, always begin with your physician. Other information about BPPV can come from many sources representing many points of view.

Chapter 17

Success Stories

The symptoms of BPPV may disappear spontaneously or after treatment. This chapter consists of stories from VEDA members whose BPPV episodes have stopped after receiving treatment specific for their condition.

Canalith Repositioning Procedure

"I am a 33-year-old woman who suffers from BPPV. I had a very severe attack in April 1995. I could not walk and had to drop out of school for the semester. This episode lasted for five months. When I became a member of VEDA, your list of doctors treating BPPV led me to a doctor in Jupiter, Fla. Your article said that this doctor performed the Epley maneuver. I set up an appointment for a consultation, and the doctor was ready to see me when I had my next attack.

"In October 1997, it happened again. I awoke to a spinning bedroom. Terrified, I called and got right in to the doctor, and with one treatment I walked out of his office with no vertigo. The vertigo never came back.

"I am so thrilled that this maneuver worked. I have a whole new outlook on life. I don't have to worry about losing my job or suffering weeks with the spinning."

—J.

"In January 1991, I had a fall. I slipped on ice and suffered a severe blow to the back of my head. Since that time, I've had recurring dizzy spells. In April 1996, I woke up to a very violent attack of dizziness. Shortly thereafter, I was diagnosed as suffering from Meniere's disease. (I suspected a virus as many of my friends had the same experience.)

"I took another fall in September; I fainted from salt depletion while on a bike. Yes, I had on a helmet but suffered a concussion. After that, the dizziness came back in full force. Looking up (top shelf) always triggered it. Some days it really knocked me out, and I had to go to bed.

"Your literature led me back to my doctor and on to the Southern Illinois School of Medicine, where I was diagnosed with BPPV and treated with the Epley maneuver. I had immediate results with only one slight reoccurrence shortly after treatment.

"Since then, I have painted the entire interior of my home (ceilings as well) and enjoy gardening, playing tennis, and riding my new bike (wearing a new helmet)."

—J.S.

Canal Plugging Surgery

"On the Saturday of Memorial Day weekend in 1992, I spent the morning planting flowers with my husband and two of my sons. Every time I stood up from kneeling in the garden, I noticed some vague symptoms of disequilibrium and queasiness, which I attributed to working in the sun on a warm and humid day. When we finished and went inside for lunch, I realized that I really did not feel very well, so I ate some lunch and decided to lie down on the couch for a nap.

"Upon awakening, I began to sit up as usual. Just raising my head caused violent dizziness with the sensation that the whole room was spinning rapidly. I was also very nauseous and realized that I had to get up because I was going to vomit, which soon happened. It was several hours before I was able to do anything but sit very still.

"This is the story of my introduction to BPPV, although it would be some time before I would make my own diagnosis thanks to a tiny 'filler' article in our local newspaper that gave the name and address for VEDA. The local ear specialist to whom I was referred had very little knowledge of vestibular disorders and preferred to spend his time on patients who were candidates for surgery. His diagnosis was chronic labyrinthitis, which I think was his way of saying he didn't know what was wrong and couldn't help me.

"For the first year or so, I had periods of relief and periods when I was seriously limited by spells of BPPV. Eventually, I reached a point where I never had a day that was symptom-free. I gradually learned which movement to avoid and which activities were on my 'no' list. I sought permission from our HMO to seek physical therapy at a local hospital and was told that they did not predict improvement from therapy, and they therefore refused coverage.

"In January of 1996, we switched to a new HMO available from the University of Michigan. I was then able to seek help at its otolaryngology clinic. They began with testing to confirm BPPV, followed by months of physical therapy, which helped a little. It enabled me to get through a normal day symptom-free as long as I did not spend a long period on my knees doing things like gardening.

"However, I am a student in a physical therapy assistant program, and I realized that I would have to change my major if I could not improve. An M.D. at the clinic told me about a surgical technique that was very successful for patients like me. The surgery involves making an opening through the temporal bone to expose the semicircular canals and then plugging the problematic canal (usually it is the posterior) with a paste made from the bone fragments. I had surgery on June 18, and I'm thrilled to report that I am cured.

"It is such a delight to be able to do things that I have avoided for years, simple things like using our weight-training equipment and pulling weeds in the garden. What a blessing."

—M.K.

References

______. *More Stories and Strategies: Coping With Vestibular Disorders*. Portland, Ore.: Vestibular Disorders Association, 1995.

Vestibular Disorders Association. *On The Level*, Fall 1997 and Winter 1998.

Appendix A:
Advanced Balance Concepts

Sending Vestibular Information

A vestibular information signal begins when gravity or acceleration bends (shears) the cilia on a hair cell. This causes secretion of a neurotransmitter (a chemical). The electrical signal created by the neurotransmitter travels in a neuron (nerve cell) along the vestibulocochlear nerve to the brain.

The sensory information goes directly to at least two areas of the brain: the vestibular nuclear complex and the cerebellum. Most of the balance information goes to the vestibular nuclear complex, also called the vestibular nuclei.

Using Vestibular Information

The information collected by the semicircular canals and otolithic organs is used for balance and some other functions including clear vision and a steady head and by the autonomic nervous system.

Balance

The movement and gravity information collected by the inner ear is sent to the vestibular nuclear complex of the brain, which uses the majority of this information immediately and reflexively. Commands are sent from this brain area to the muscles in the neck, trunk, arms, and legs via the vestibulo-spinal reflex (VSR) and the vestibular-collic reflex (VCR). The muscle changes or adjustments necessary to stay upright and move around safely are then carried out.

Definition: Balance is defined by *Stedman's Medical Dictionary* as a state of repose between two or more antagonistic forces that exactly counteract each other. With relation to human balance, this generally means using your muscles to counteract gravity and other forces by keeping your center of gravity aligned properly over your feet.

Clear Vision, Steady Head

Vision and the vestibular system work together to enhance visual accuracy via the VOR. Vestibular information is used to reposition your eyes during movement involving the head. This repositioning keeps your eyes fixed on whatever you are looking at. If your eyes did not move appropriately, things in your field of vision would appear to bounce when you moved your head.

The VCR also helps to keep your eyes directed at what you are looking at by using movement and gravity information to position your head rapidly. In addition, the VCR works to keep your head steady and in an appropriate position, usually vertical.

Autonomic Adjustments

A number of automatic body functions, including blood pressure, are regulated by the autonomic nervous system (ANS). The ANS uses vestibular information to institute immediate changes in these body functions to maintain a normal or healthy internal environment.

For example, if no immediate changes in blood vessel diameter occurred when you stood up, your blood pressure would drop and you might feel lightheaded. Vestibular information keeps the blood pressure stable in the first milliseconds of a position change, allowing time for the other regulatory mechanisms to kick in.

Systems Involved in Balance

Balance is not maintained purely by information from the vestibular parts of the inner ear. Many factors are required, and two other systems, vision and proprioception, come into play.

Table A-1: Conditions Required for Normal Balance

- Your inner ears must be functioning normally.
- Your brain (cerebrum, cerebellum, and brain stem) must be functioning properly.
- You must be awake and alert.
- Your spinal cord must be working.
- Your muscle strength must be adequate, especially the leg and trunk muscles.
- Your joints must have adequate flexibility, particularly the ankles, knees, and hips.

The best, most efficient balance occurs when all the factors are in place and the three systems continuously contribute their information to balance. However, if one system is lost, the other two can provide enough information for you to move around within limitations after you practice. Even so, depending too much on vision or proprioception for balance can create new problems.

Definition: Proprioception is information about gravity, position, surfaces, and stretch and motion of the muscles and joints that is collected by the system of pressure sensors scattered around the skeletal muscles, tendons, joints, ligaments, and connective tissue covering the bones and muscles. This information is used to determine what movement is being undertaken and where different body parts are in relationship to one another. You need proprioception to find the tip of your nose with your finger when your eyes are closed, for example.

Vision

Vision contributes quite a bit to balance. It helps you to avoid obstacles. Vision assists in balance by helping to determine how your body is moving with respect to objects in your environment. For example, if you move forward, objects you are looking at grow larger on your retina, while objects you are moving away from appear to shrink. With vision, you can tell if only your head is moving or if the movement includes your entire body. Vision can detect constant movement not sensed by the vestibular apparatus. It can sense the direction and speed of movement. Vision can help determine where vertical and horizontal are and if you are "straight" or leaning to the side.

The problem with primarily using vision for balance is that it is ambiguous and allows the brain to think there is movement when there is none. Busy patterns on carpets, curtains, or wall paper; stripes on a crosswalk (zebra crossing); movement across a TV or movie screen, or just moving the eyes can all increase the ambiguity. Without normal vestibular function, you can be constantly fooled into thinking that either you or things near you are moving.

An example of being fooled by vision is called a "vection illusion." If you have ever felt as if you were moving because the car next to you was moving, you have experienced vection illusion. This feeling can be so strong that you will suddenly push harder on your car's foot brake even though you were already braking. This is a "normal" experience if it lasts only a second or so in an otherwise normal environment.

Proprioception

Proprioception also contributes a lot of necessary information for balance. This system senses the stress in the muscles. During standing, the stress is caused by the force of gravity, which will pull your weight to the ground if your muscles do not contract. Some of the most important proprioceptors are in the neck. These receptors give the brain additional input to determine if your entire body is moving or if only your head is moving.

Vision and proprioception supply information the vestibular apparatus is unable to get, and they also collect partially duplicated information. Thus the "system" for collecting balance information is redundant when all three systems are working properly.

Balance Factors

Because of the redundancy or duplication of information, with practice you can stand upright and walk without vestibular input if you are not in a visually confusing situation and you are walking on a firm surface.

Successful balance ability, when you are up and about, depends upon how you are able to use your muscles during different situations. The way your brain responds to situations requiring adjustments to maintain balance depends not only on the information collected by the inner ears and other sensory inputs but also on your muscles and their attached nerves. Your motor (movement) response to changing situations depends upon your expectations, experience, and practice.

When you know what to expect, your brain is better able to make the necessary adjustments. For example, if you are subjected to several series of identical changes, you learn what to expect and make rapid and accurate adjustments. If, on the other hand, you are subjected to a series of random changes, your adjustments will not be as rapid or accurate.

Experience with different situations is also something that can enhance balance. For example, your first few attempts at riding a bicycle were probably not successful. At some point you "got it," that is, you experienced a moment of balance on two wheels, and after that you "understood" what you needed to do. This kind of knowledge cannot be gained by watching someone else ride a bicycle or by being told what two-wheeled riding is like. Once you experience balance under cycling conditions, you keep the experience in your brain, and you can revisit it even after years of not riding a bicycle. Returning to a bicycle after years of being away is easy compared to learning to ride the first time.

Practice, performing an activity over and over, improves balance in that activity and usually results in improvement. For example, trying to change the swing of an experienced baseball player or golfer will usually result initially in a slow, stiff, uneasy swing. With many repetitions, the swing will feel and look natural (and may improve the batting average or golf score).

More on Vision

As odd as it probably sounds, the eyes are closely linked to the ears, and they depend upon each other for good balance and clear vision. The relationship is a two-way street; the ears help you to see clearly, and the eyes help with your balance. This link is the scientific basis for a good deal of the current, sophisticated vestibular testing like rotary testing, caloric testing (part of an ENG), and computerized dynamic posturography. (For more on these tests, see Appendix C, "More About Tests") It is also the reason some people with BPPV experience uncomfortable symptoms involving the eyes and vision.

Nerve cells (neurons) link the inner ears to the eyes. Each hair cell of the vestibular end organs requires only three neurons to link it via other structures to the muscles that move the eyes. This link carries messages and commands from the inner ears to the eyes via the brain.

The movement and gravity information collected by the vestibular areas of the ear travels to the vestibular area of the brain along the first neuron. The second neuron transmits this information to the brain area that controls eye movement. The third neuron carries commands from the eye movement area of the brain to the muscles attached to the outside of the eye, and the commands cause eye movement. This lightning-quick chain of events is referred to as the vestibulo-ocular reflex or VOR.

The VOR is different from many reflex systems because the brain can change VOR information. This difference helps to maintain clear vision under the greatest number of conditions but also makes its function more complicated and difficult to explain or understand.

When you move your head, the VOR uses vestibular information to adjust your eyes smoothly in the direction opposite to which your head is moving. Not only do the eyes move in a direction precisely opposite to the head movement, they do so at the same time and at the same speed as the head movement. Without this action, your eyes would be in a fixed position with respect to your head during movements like walking, running, and driving, and the world would appear to be bouncing up and down with each step or bump in the road. The look would be similar to the bouncing picture an inexperienced camera operator might shoot with a video camera.

The "seeing" part of the eye is the retina, located at the back of the eye. To clearly see an object and keep seeing it while you move, the image of the object must be kept still on the back of the eye.

Rotation testing is a convenient way for doctors to determine how well the VOR is working. The speed and timing of the eye movement response are analyzed to determine if they are within the normal range.

References

Alexander, N.B. "Postural Control in Older Adults." *Journal of the American Geriatric Society*, 42(1):93-108, 1994.

Keshner, E.A., and Cohen, H. "Current Concepts of the Vestibular System Reviewed: 1. The Role of the Vestibulospinal System in Postural Control." *American Journal of Occupational Therapy*, 43:331-337, 1989.

Sharpe, J.A., and Barber, H.O. *The Vestibulo-Ocular Reflex and Vertigo*. New York: Raven Press, 1993.

Wilson, V.J., Boyle, R., Fukushima, K., Rose, P.K., Shinoda, Y., Sugiuchi, Y., and Uchino, Y. "The Vestibulocollic Reflex." *Journal of Vestibular Research*, 5(3):147-170, 1995.

Yates, B.J. and Miller, S.D. *Vestibular Autonomic Regulation*. Boca Raton, Florida: CRC Press, Inc., 1996.

Appendix B:

Possible Symptoms of Severe/Persistent BPPV

Table B-1:
Symptoms That Might Occur in Persistent or Extreme BPPV
(There are not specific to BPPV. They can result from other vestibular disorders as well.)

General feelings
Disconnection
Drunkenness
Fatigue
Hangover
Malaise
Seasickness
Spaciness

Head Sensations
Floating
Headache
Lightheadedness
Motion sickness
Swimming

Emotions
Anger/rage
Anxiety
Depression
Fear
Loss of self-confidence
Loss of self-esteem
Loss of self-reliance
Worry

Movement/Walking
Awkwardness
Clumsiness
Difficulty turning
Feeling of impending backwards falling
Groping for stable objects
Imbalance
Motion intolerance
Need to look down while walking
Need to touch things while walking
Staggering
Stumbling
Sudden falls
Unsteadiness
Walking-on-pillow sensation

Muscles
Neck ache
Stiff neck
Stiffness
Trembling

Spatial Orientation
Dizziness
Sense of floating
Sense of tilt
Spatial disorientation

Thought
Difficulty concentrating
Distractibility
Groping for words

Vision
Blurred vision
Difficulty looking through binoculars, cameras, microscopes, telescopes and similar things
Difficulty watching movement
Focusing problems
Jumping vision
Reading problems

Note: Symptoms not associated with vestibular disorders that should be reported immediately to your physician include the following:

- weakness (such as an inability to raise an arm or leg or to clench a fist)
- numbness
- loss of vision (partial or total)
- inability to speak, loss of voice
- sudden loss of hearing
- loss of consciousness
- difficulty swallowing

Hangover, Malaise

A disruption in the vestibular system affects much more than your balance. Vestibular information is needed not only for balance but also for clear vision and some autonomic nervous system functions.

When your vestibular function is normal, you balance automatically. If you have a severe form of BPPV, you will have to think more often about balance to maintain it. Your brain may struggle (consciously and unconsciously) to adjust during episodes of vertigo and may continue to struggle after the vertigo stops. As vestibular signals return to normal, your brain will re-adjust, and your symptoms will fade until the next episode of vertigo. If your episodes come frequently with little time between, your brain may be unable to fully re-adjust.

The consequence of disruption in vestibular signals can include lightheadedness, fatigue, malaise, and other symptoms listed in Table B-1. The hangover feelings can include fatigue, headache, a desire to avoid other people, sensitivity to lights and sounds, a queasy stomach, and overreaction when surprised. These sensations can feel similar to an alcohol hangover, which is not surprising because alcohol directly affects the inner ear. In fact, the inner ear may produce the alcohol hangover or at least parts of it.

Unsteadiness

When your brain receives inconsistent vestibular information and tries to adjust, movement can be an adventure. Staggering, stumbling, clumsiness, awkwardness, and unsteadiness can occur. It will be more pronounced when you can't see, either in the dark or when your eyes are closed.

Unsteadiness can occur when inappropriate movement signals are sent to the brain and cause problems with the vestibular reflexes.

Some people with BPPV stand and/or walk with their feet further apart than usual in an effort, conscious or unconscious, to prevent falling. A wider base creates more stability.

"Unsteady" can describe how you look as you move, or it can describe how you feel. You can feel unsteady without looking unsteady.

Stiff Muscles, Inflexible Joints

Muscles of the neck, trunk, arms and legs can become stiff, sometimes to the point of trembling. Normal muscle movements require normal vestibular reflexes. If your vestibular reflexes are not normal, your neck muscles and muscles used for upright movement will not contract and relax normally. You may feel awkward when you move and may suffer later from sore muscles.

During an episode of BPPV, your neck muscles may become automatically rigid to prevent head movement and the worsening of symptoms. In trying to prevent vertigo, these muscles may become stiff when you move about or try to move your head, particularly into positions that have caused problems before.

Some people with BPPV stop their normal activities and severely limit their movement to prevent a worsening of symptoms. This can lead to reduced muscle strength and reduced joint flexibility that in turn produce unsteadiness and other balance problems.

> "Patients who are untreated often limit their daily activities . . . to prevent onset of vertigo. In some cases this limiting of daily activities can result in loss of ROM (range of motion—the ability to move the extremities and other body parts as far as they should be able to move) in the neck, trunk and legs; decrease in job performance, and delay recovery from vertigo."
>
> —C. D. Ford-Smith, P.T., *Physical Therapy*, 1997

Impaired Cognition

"My thinking was definitely impaired on my bad days. In my writing, I would leave off the first letter in a word. It was as if I had a learning disability."

—V.N., letter to the author, 1998

When your BPPV is active, you might experience lack of concentration, distraction, groping for words, decreased ability to reason, trouble with judgment, writing difficulty, and poor memory. Some people may even stutter. The reasons for this are not well understood. They might be related to the brainwork required to maintain balance despite BPPV. Disrupted sleep, particularly if it is frequent, may also cause these symptoms.

Negative Emotions

Fear and anxiety are common when vertigo hits. They may persist because you are thinking about the next episode of vertigo and how BPPV is damaging your life.

These symptoms can be distracting and disturbing to the point of causing dread, that something else even more serious is actually happening (such as a stroke, brain tumor, heart attack, going crazy). These thoughts can lead to more worry, fear, and anxiety.

"I feel angry and fearful and resentful."

—V.H., letter to the author, 1998

If the BPPV is present for long, it may change the way you view yourself and the way you live. This can cause anger or depression.

The vertigo and other symptoms, in some people, may come so frequently that they drastically affect how these people live. Needing medical advice and care and being forced to ask other people for daily help can be severely disruptive. Productive, self-sufficient people may lose their self-reliance, self-confidence, and self-esteem because they are no longer able to live as independently as in the past.

Disturbed Vision

"When my BPPV is in an active phase, I tend to have problems with depth perception and judging distances and will often cut corners too closely, running into door jambs with my right arm or shoulder."

—S.P., letter to the author, 1998

Visual problems can affect focusing, reading, and looking at moving objects, and may involve blurring and distortion.

If your vestibular information is no longer accurate because of BPPV, you will rely more heavily on vision than normal to maintain your balance. This dependence on vision will make you more vulnerable than normal to conditions of reduced or distorted vision. You will notice more symptoms during low-light conditions or in places such as crowded stadiums, theaters, and supermarkets with complex, dynamic visual activity. Looking at moving objects may trigger nausea and dizziness. Scanning a line of type in a book or looking at screen scrolling on a computer may cause similar problems.

Headache

Headaches can result from general malaise, as a part of a hangover effect, from muscle strain from trying to focus your eyes, or from holding your head rigidly to prevent vertigo.

References

Epley, J.M. "New Dimensions of Benign Paroxysmal Positional Vertigo." *Otolaryngology- Head and Neck Surgery,* 88:599-605, 1980.

Ford-Smith, C.D. "The Individualized Treatment of a Patient with Benign Paroxysmal Positional Vertigo." *Physical Therapy,* 77(8):848-855, 1997.

Potter, P.A., and Perry, A.G. *Basic Nursing: Theory and Practice.* St. Louis: Mosby. 1995.

Schuknecht, H.F. "Cupulolithiasis." *Archives of Otolaryngology-Head and Neck Surgery,* 90:113-126, 1969.

Appendix C:
More About Tests

Basic Testing Concepts

Most disorders of the inner ear can be difficult to test for because the inner ear is tiny and embedded within the densest bone of the body. The interior of the inner ear can't be seen or visualized with currently available technology (ultrasound, X-ray, CT scan, MRI). The inner ear also cannot be entered with any instrument without risking loss of hearing and vestibular function. Therefore neither normal function nor abnormal function can be seen directly.

As you read the following information about testing, keep in mind that VEDA and this author do not mean to endorse or disavow the tests described here. We're not suggesting that all these tests be performed to diagnose BPPV or to rule out (exclude) other conditions. We're describing the examination and tests to help explain what they measure, what they're like, and for what reasons (other then diagnosis) they might be used. VEDA and the author are not suggesting the use of one or another of the tests in a particular situation. We have included the following descriptions because the doctors of some people with BPPV may order tests in addition to those reviewed in Chapter 6.

Allergy note: Many of these tests use "sticky patches," electrodes that are stuck to the body, usually on the face and/or head. They usually contain water, glycerol, and polyacrylic acid (containing sodium sulfonate groups). If you are allergic to any of these, notify your doctor's office and the testing center.

Test Categories

Tests given to people with vestibular disorders can be divided into three categories: tests of hearing, tests of vestibular function, and miscellaneous tests. Hearing is measured "directly," and balance function is mostly measured "indirectly." The tests of vestibular function may be referred to as balance tests, but most observe or measure eye movement. Because of the vestibular-ocular reflex, the eyes are something of a window on the inner ear.

The goals of the tests are to:

- Decide if the problem is in the ear or elsewhere.
- Determine the side or sides involved.
- Rule out the presence of a tumor or other serious neurological problems.

If your doctor wants you to undergo tests beyond those specific to BPPV, you might ask the following questions:

- Do I need these tests?
- What do these other tests look at or for?
- Are any risks or dangers involved? If risk is involved, do alternatives exist?

If you have questions about your testing, try to discuss them with your doctor or your doctor's staff. The audiologist may be able to answer your questions. These professionals are the only ones who can tell you why they did or did not request a certain test and what the results mean in your particular case. If for some reason you feel under-tested and belong to an HMO or other managed care arrangement, ask the doctor if any tests have been left out solely at the request of the insurance company or to save money. Don't assume you would be told this if it was a factor.

Note about insurance: If you are with an HMO (health maintenance organization), don't go for a test unless you have the proper referral. If you are with a PPO (preferred provider organization), make sure the doctor or testing place is on the approved list. Sometimes a chat beforehand with the billing clerk at your doctor's office or the testing center can alert you to potential insurance problems.

No available tests can "see" inside the vestibular apparatus or directly measure the balance information going to the brain via the vestibulo-cochlear nerve. The tests can't directly determine if the vestibular apparatus is working normally. However, tests can investigate vestibular function indirectly by looking at two reflexes that depend on vestibular information. These reflexes are called the vestibulo-ocular reflex (VOR) and the vestibulo-spinal reflex (VSR). The available tests look at the function of the VOR and that of the VSR and provide indirect methods of checking on vestibular function.

Health professionals often review results of hearing tests when establishing a diagnosis of BPPV. BPPV itself does not cause hearing problems, but other inner ear diseases that may accompany or cause BPPV can cause hearing problems.

Vestibular Function Tests

Only the Dix-Hallpike test can document BPPV of the posterior and/or anterior canals, and sometimes doctors will try a similar test to try to document the horizontal canal variant. In addition, your doctor may order other tests of the vestibular system to determine its general condition and to exclude other causes of your symptoms. These tests include electronystagmography, rotation testing, and computerized dynamic posturography

Electronystagmography (ENG)

"ENG" is a label commonly used improperly in referring to a group or battery of eye movement tests that look for signs of vestibular dysfunction or neurological problems. This common use is inaccurate because not all ENG tests involve nystagmus (abnormal eye jerking), and the health professionals who conduct these tests often use them to measure eye movements other than nystagmus. However, because the tests are so commonly referred to as "an ENG," we will do so to avoid confusion.

ENG tests are probably the most common of the tests administered to people with dizziness, vertigo, and/or balance disorders, but neither the test battery nor the testing method is standardized.

Insurance/billing note: If you receive itemized medical bills for this test battery, you will probably find a list of different tests. The initials "ENG" most likely will not appear on the bill.

An ENG can include the following tests:

- visual tracking (can also be called visual-ocular control, ocular dysmetria testing)
- optokinetic nystagmus
- optokinetic after-nystagmus
- saccades testing
- smooth pursuit
- spontaneous nystagmus
- gaze
- positional
- positioning (Dix-Hallpike). See Chapter 6.
- fistula or pressure testing
- head shaking
- caloric (may also be called bithermal caloric, monothermal caloric)

Special Instruction

Blinking interferes with test interpretation. Try to avoid blinking during an ENG test.

What It Is Like

The test and its preparation generally require at least 60 minutes. First, areas around your eyes will be cleaned and sticky-patch electrodes applied so that your eye movements can be electrically monitored. See Figure C-1 for an example.

During this test, the person in charge will give you many instructions. You may be asked to follow this or that with your eyes, stare at something, move your eyes from here to there, close your eyes, open your eyes, turn your head, roll on your side, or count backwards from 100 by threes.

You will be asked to move into different positions from sitting up to lying down on one side or another or turning your head to one side or another. Most of these position changes are slow except for the "Dix-Hallpike" or positioning test. (See Chapter 6.)

During the fistula or pressure test, an earplug will be placed in the external auditory canal of one ear, through which positive and nega-

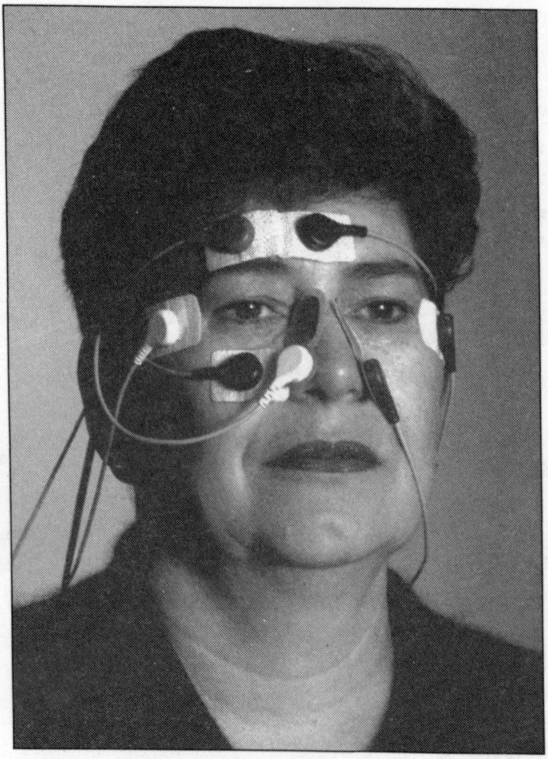

Figure C-1: Sticky-patch electrodes. A woman prepared for ENG testing. (Courtesy of Micromedical Technologies, Chatham, Illinois.)

tive pressure will be introduced while your eye movement is measured. The tester will test one ear at a time.

The caloric test is generally done last. The majority of people having an ENG find this test to be the most uncomfortable and memorable because it can cause temporary vertigo accompanied by nausea.

The most commonly administered caloric test has four parts and is called the bithermal alternating caloric. The temperature in the external auditory canal of each ear is temporarily changed by a few degrees a total of four times (first ear warm, second ear warm, first ear cool, second ear cool). Your tester will probably slide a catheter into your ear canal to deliver air or water to induce the temperature change. The reaction of the eyes (nystagmus) to this change will be measured while you perform a mental task such as counting backwards from 100 by subtracting threes or naming things starting with a certain letter.

Note: Some physicians change the temperature in both ears simultaneously instead of the more standard alternation method, and others change the temperature only once rather than twice.

The temperature change causes a spinning sensation, which is most intense about 60 seconds into the test. The strength of the spinning depends upon the amount of vestibular function present.

A normal ear will produce the greatest spinning response. Absence of spinning during this part of the test indicates that vestibular function is absent on the side being tested. If this occurs, the tester may retry the test with ice water.

At some point after the entire temperature change has occurred, you will be asked to fix your vision on something straight ahead, such as a red light or a dot on the ceiling. This visual fixation will stop the nystagmus and spinning caused by the temperature change. This procedure will be repeated for each of the four parts of the test.

Note: Some testing centers use infrared goggles instead of sticky patch electrodes. When you are tested with goggles, you will be asked to keep your eyes open throughout the test. The goggles look a bit like ski goggles and are a bit more comfortable than electrodes. Unlike the electrode method, the goggle method doesn't rely on recording the electricity generated by eye movement. Instead, this computerized test "sees" the eyes during the test and can detect any movement, including rotary and vertical, not just horizontal.

What These Tests Show

All tests except the Dix-Hallpike should be normal in anyone with posterior BPPV unaccompanied by other vestibular problems. If a reduced response to caloric testing is found, it tells your doctor that a problem exists either with the horizontal canal or the vestibulo-cochlear nerve on the tested side, or with the brain. A reduced response is also sometimes found in the horizontal canal variant of BPPV.

In some cases, eye movement tests can indicate a brain problem rather than an inner ear problem or vice versa. Certain types of nystagmus come from specific areas of the brain; their presence will point to a problem in those areas. Sometimes the ENG does not reveal any problems, but unfortunately this does not rule out the possibility of BPPV.

Other Uses

Like the hearing test, the ENG test battery may be used to periodically monitor your condition if you have a vestibular problem in addition to BPPV.

After the Test

This test can cause nausea, fatigue, and a temporary off-balance sensation. Plan to have someone drive you home from the test, or allow enough time to recover before driving.

Rotational Testing

Rotational or turning tests cannot diagnose BPPV but can be helpful in identifying other vestibular problems. Rotational tests examine the vestibulo-ocular reflex (VOR). These tests may be passive or active. During a passive test, you are moved by a machine or by another person. During an active test, you move yourself.

Rotary Chair

One of these tests, the rotary chair test, may also be called SHAT or SHA for "sinusoidal harmonic acceleration test." This is a computerized, passive, objective test of the horizontal VOR.

The SHAT may also be referred to as total body rotational testing. One property of the VOR is that when vision is absent (in darkness or with the eyes closed), turning the head in one direction normally results in simultaneous movement of the eyes at exactly the same speed in the opposite direction. The rotary chair test is designed to examine this property.

What It Is Like

The test is done in a small room, where you sit in a motor-driven computerized chair with your head flexed forward a bit and the lights turned off. Before beginning the test, the person in charge of the test will clean areas of your face, apply electrodes to the clean areas, and put headphones on you to enable constant contact with the tester outside the room. The test and its preparation generally require 40 to 45 minutes.

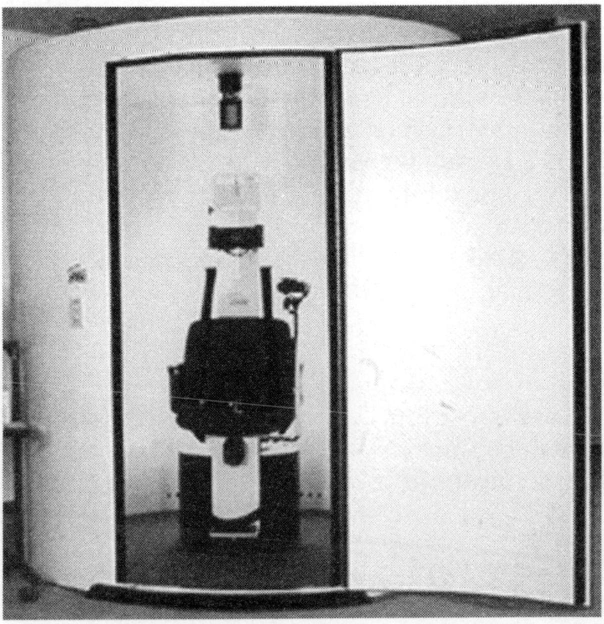

Figure C-2: Rotary chair. (Courtesy of Micromedical Technologies, Chatham, Illinois.)

The test itself has two general parts, chair movement and visual testing. The chair usually moves slowly back and forth through 180 degrees, not around in a full circle. During chair movement, you will not be asked to participate in any way other than to speak to the tester at times. (In a few testing centers, the chair movement is faster.) During the visual gaze section, you will be asked to find and follow a little red light with your eyes. Some testing places also add another part, the optokinetic drum test, with the room lights on.

What It Shows

The rotary chair test shows how well the central nervous system is processing vestibular information and how well the brain integrates visual/vestibular information. This test shows how the VOR is working and how well you can fix your vision on something. Your doctor wants to know if your eyes move at the same speed as the movement of the chair and how long it takes for your eyes to move once the chair moves.

The test can, at times, show the presence of a vestibular problem but does not usually help identify which ear has the problem because both sides are stimulated simultaneously. No rotary chair result by itself specifically identifies BPPV.

After the Test

This test should not have any long-term effect on you or your vestibular symptoms. If movement aggravates your symptoms, plan to have someone drive you home from the test, or allow enough time to stay at the testing center until your symptoms resolve.

Comparison

The rotary chair test requires a computerized moving chair in its own special little room. The test is done at a slower speed than the other two rotational tests (the HSVOR and head-only auto-rotational testing described below). During the test, your head and body move as a unit; your head does not rotate alone, and it is passive rather than active. The rotary chair test is more similar from clinic to clinic than the ENG battery. Many people find the rotary chair test easier and more comfortable than caloric testing.

Other Uses

The SHAT can be used to assess how the brain is "compensating" for a permanent loss of vestibular function and can be used over time to look at this phenomenon. Sometimes it is also used over time to assess how someone is doing and is a good test for assessing people with bilateral losses.

Head-Shaking Test (HSVOR)

Another rotational test, the head-shaking test is also called the head-shaking vestibulo-ocular reflex test or HSVOR. It is usually a non-computerized, passive test. (Someone will move your head for you.)

What It Is Like

The HSVOR is done while you sit, usually wearing Frenzel lenses. The tester moves your head back and forth with his or her hands and observes your eyes for nystagmus.

What It Shows

This test produces nystagmus, the speed and direction of which are observed and sometimes recorded. An abnormal test can suggest a problem with the vestibulo-ocular reflex, either in the inner ear, the vestibular nerve, or the brain. No specific HSVOR result establishes the presence of BPPV.

After the Test

Although it can cause temporary fatigue and a feeling of imbalance, this test should not have any long-term effect on you or your symptoms. If movement aggravates your symptoms, plan to have someone drive you home from the test, or stay at the testing center until they resolve.

Auto-Rotational Testing

A third type of rotational test, the auto-rotational test, is computerized. It measures your ability to keep your eyes focused on a stationary target during active head movement, both back and forth and up and down. The test is also referred to as a head-on-body rotation test, a head-only auto-rotational test, or an active head rotation test, or may be identified by a proprietary name —vestibular auto-rotation test (VAT) or vestibulo-ocular reflex testing equipment (VORTEQ) test. It can test the VOR both horizontally and vertically.

What It Is Like

Electrodes are placed on your face to measure eye movement, and a device resembling a band is placed around your head to measure the speed of any head movement. (See Figure C-3.) While in a sitting position, you are asked to move your head back and forth in time with a sound for no longer than 18 seconds while looking at a visual target (usually a dot) close by. This visual target may appear to jump during the test, but it actually remains stationary. The procedure is repeated twice more at different speeds and then, after a short pause, you will be asked to repeat the performance substituting up-and-down movements for back-and-forth movements. This test requires about 20 minutes including preparation time.

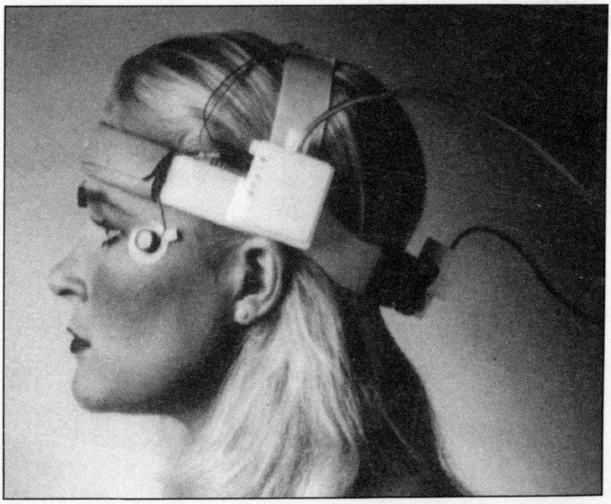

Figure C-3: Vestibular auto-rotation test (VAT). (Courtesy of Western Systems Research, Pasadena California.)

What It Shows

This test shows how well you keep your eyes fixed on a stationary target while your head is moving. To keep your vision trained on a stationary target while moving your head, you must move your eyes. It is this eye movement that is recorded and studied.

An abnormal test result shows a problem with the VOR. Recent studies with the VAT indicate that a specific test result may indicate the presence of posterior canal BPPV.

Comparisons

Auto-rotation testing does not require a dedicated room or computerized "furniture" like the SHAT (rotary chair test). (It should be billed at a lower price.) Auto-rotation testing studies both horizontal and vertical head movement and also studies the VOR at higher speeds (which is probably more like the movement encountered in everyday life) than the rotary chair test. Auto-rotation testing is done quickly compared to most other vestibular tests. Many people consider it more comfortable than ENG testing.

After the Test

People sensitive to head movement or eye movement after head movement may have their symptoms temporarily stirred up by this test. Plan to have someone drive you home, or stay put until you are able to drive.

Computerized Dynamic Posturography (CDP)

This is a group of tests of the vestibulo-spinal reflex (VSR), which creates muscle movements necessary to maintain balance when you are standing or sitting. Computerized dynamic posturography (CDP) is also sometimes called dynamic posturography, moving platform posturography, dynamic computerized platform posturography, and platform posturography. A computer creates the changing conditions you experience during the test and automatically records your body's responses.

Preparation

Because the testing equipment includes a harness to keep you from falling, wear shorts or slacks for the test. You will also be asked to remove your shoes and possibly your socks. Allow about an hour for the test.

Insurance/billing note: Some insurance companies will not pay for CDP testing. Check with your insurance company before scheduling the test. The testing center may also be able to give you a general idea about problems related to insurance. If you receive itemized bills, CDP testing may be charged in two or three parts: sensory organization test, motor coordination test, and pressure test.

What It Is Like

Before beginning the test, you will be fitted with a harness similar to those worn by parachutists or rock climbers. (See Figure C-4.) It will keep you from falling down if you lose your balance. You will be asked to stand quietly on a flat surface during the entire test and will be given instructions about when to open your eyes and when to close them. The surface under your feet will be still at times and will move at other times. The "wall" directly in front of you will be still and perfectly vertical at most times but will automatically move slightly at times. Sometimes a pressure test will be included in CDP testing. It involves inserting an earpiece, introducing positive and negative pressure, and measuring your movement or sway. This procedure is repeated with positive and negative pressure in each ear, one ear at a time.

What It Shows

CDP testing shows how well you maintain balance in response to various situations, such as when information is available from vision, proprioception, and the vestibular apparatus vs. when information is available from only two or only one of these systems or when the information from one or more is inaccurate. Information is unavailable or inaccurate when your eyes are closed, when the "wall" is moving, and when the surface under your feet is allowed to move.

Testing also measures muscle response to changing balance situations. You use certain muscle "strategies" subconsciously and automatically to maintain balance, and these can also be assessed.

Finally, CDP can measure balance response to increased and decreased pressure in each ear. CDP can indicate if a problem is present but not whether the trouble is in the inner ear, nerve, or brain. A possible exception is pressure testing done one ear at a time; presumably, the pressure can affect only the middle ear and inner ear windows on the side being tested. Studies indicate that people with BPPV have abnormal CDP test results and may rely disproportionately on vision or proprioception and not enough on vestibular information. However, no generally accepted CDP result specifically identifies BPPV.

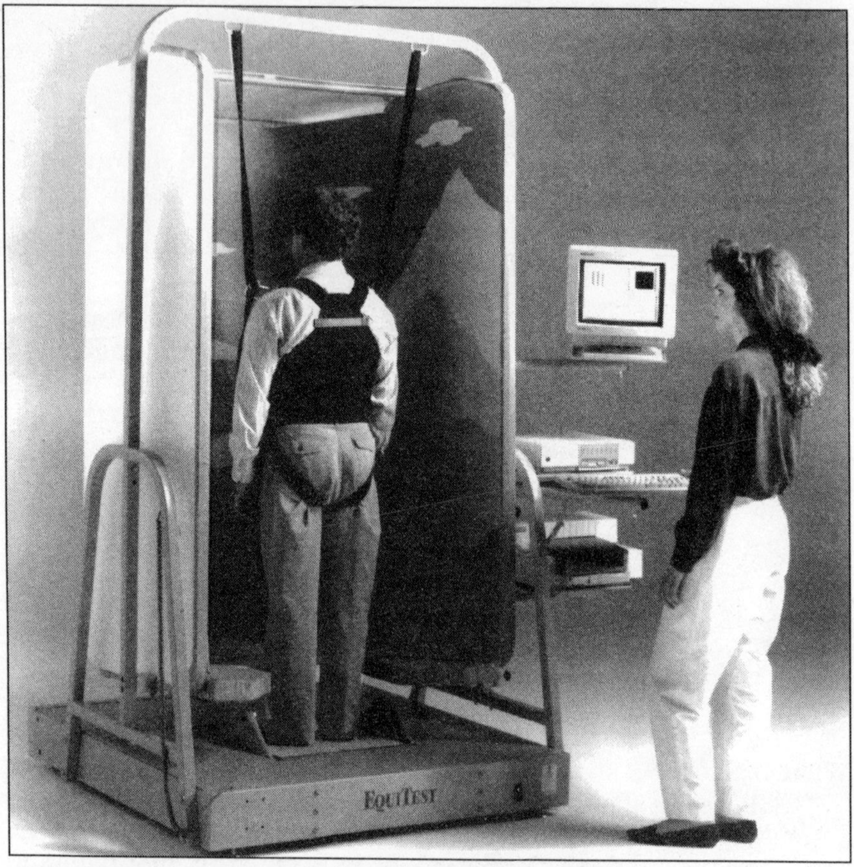

Figure 16-5: Computerized dynamic posturography. (Courtesy of NeuroCom International, Inc., Clackamas, Oregon.)

Other Uses

Because this test shows muscle responses, some doctors use it not only to help make a diagnosis but to determine if some type of physical therapy might help you and, if so, what type.

The test can also be repeated from time to time to document changes in balance ability.

Comparisons

CDP is different from the other tests because it is done standing, does not use facial electrodes, tests body movement rather than eye movement, and usually involves no mental tasking or exercises. This test is the only computerized test discussed in this chapter that does not measure the VOR. Instead it looks at the VSR and the muscle movement it produces. CDP can also be used to develop specific physical therapy exercises that could be of benefit.

After the Test

CDP should not cause any ill effects other than momentary spatial disorientation, confusion about your position in space, and possibly some fatigue. If this test sounds like something that would bother you, ask someone to drive you home from the test, or stay put until you are again able to drive.

Tests of Hearing

Tests of hearing require no preparation or instructions beforehand. Just show up on time and follow any instructions given by the audiologist. Since you must consciously participate in the tests, go as rested and as relaxed as you can.

To check middle ear function, the audiologist will insert a plug into the external auditory canal of the ear to be tested. Via the plug, a computer will automatically increase and decrease air pressure to the ear and measure the ability of the tympanic membrane to move. This is done one ear at a time and should be painless.

The hearing tests are done in a soundproof booth using headphones to assure that the only things you can hear are the audiologist and the test sounds. Both sounds and speech are used. A series of tones at several pitches (also called frequencies) are presented to each ear. You are asked to respond when you hear the tone by raising your hand or pressing a button, and the audiologist determines at what loudness (also called decibel level) you heard it. Sometimes, in addition to the pure tones, a sound similar to radio static, called masking, is used.

Another part of the hearing tests determines how well you recognize spoken words (speech discrimination) and at what decibel level (speech reception threshold) you can understand them. The audiologist will ask you to repeat each word he or she says or perhaps will play a tape with words to repeat. Your speech discrimination will be recorded as the percentage of single syllable words that you successfully repeat. Your speech reception threshold will be the loudness or decibel level at which you can understand half of the equally weighted two-syllable words well enough to repeat them successfully. ("Baseball" is an example of a two-syllable equal-weight word.)

What the Tests Show

If a hearing loss is present, the tests will show at what frequency it occurs, at what decibel level, and whether it involves the middle ear or the cochlea/nerve/brain. The tests will also reveal speech discrimination ability; that is, how well speech is understood, and whether the speech discrimination score is consistent with the level of hearing.

ABR

The ABR is a sophisticated, computerized test of hearing. As sound makes its way to the brainstem (a part of the brain), it creates an electrical signal. This signal is recorded during the ABR and analyzed. The ABR is also referred to as a "brainstem elicited response" that may be abbreviated as BER, BSER, BAER, and so on. The test is usually referred to as an *auditory brainstem response* by otolaryngologists and as a *brainstem elicited response* by neurologists.

What It Is Like

The test is done in a quiet area while you are comfortably seated or reclining. Sticky patches (electrodes) are placed on your head. You are asked to rest quietly while listening to the sounds introduced by headphones. You are not asked to respond.

What It Shows

If hearing is abnormal, the ABR shows where in the pathway the problem lies. Under certain circumstances, this test can indicate the presence of a tumor called an acoustic neuroma. Before the advent of the MRI, this was the only test for acoustic neuroma (a benign tumor of the vestibular branch of the vestibulo-cochlear nerve).

Other Uses

Some doctors use the ABR to look for a condition sometimes called vascular compression.

MRI

In some ways a magnetic resonance imaging (MRI) scan is similar to an X-ray since you are expected to be still during the test and since the final product looks like an X-ray image. But there is one big difference: an MRI uses a magnetic field instead of X-rays.

A brain MRI is not used to "find" BPPV; it is used to look for brain abnormalities such as those caused by multiple sclerosis, stroke, and tumors. Some brain abnormalities can, on very rare occasion, cause symptoms similar to those of BPPV. Some doctors request an MRI almost automatically for people with vertigo, while others do so only if the symptoms and medical history point strongly toward the possibility of a brain problem or if standard BPPV treatments fail to help.

Preparation

Before scheduling or going for an MRI, get written instructions from the staff of your doctor's office or the testing center and read them carefully. If you have any metal in your body, you must discuss this with the testing staff. Metal would include a cardiac pacemaker, orthopedic "pin," a Cody tack, shrapnel, coronary artery clips, any type of vascular clips, a vena caval umbrella, joint prosthesis, neurostimulator, orthodontics, insulin infusion pump, middle ear prosthesis, bullets, or small bits of metal that a metal worker might have picked up through his or her career. (The testing center should provide you with a more complete list of possible body metals.) If you have some type of medical implant, do not assume that anyone else knows about it. Ask and inform.

If you are prone to claustrophobia, discuss it with your doctor or the staff of the testing center. Some MRI machines are designed in an "open" fashion, but most of them are of the older, "closed" variety.

Special Precautions

This test cannot be stopped midway without interfering with the brain image it is creating. Use the restroom before beginning the test to avoid the problems a test stoppage would create.

Do not enter the MRI room with computer disks, an ATM card, debit card, or anything else with a magnetic coded strip on the back. The magnetic field will erase all these things.

How It Works

This testing method is used to see soft tissue (not bones) using a large magnetic field instead of traditional X-rays. The magnetic field causes the hydrogen ions of the body to change position; this causes the ions to give off radio waves. A receiver detects the radio waves and sends information to a computer, which constructs an image.

What It Is Like

You will be asked to arrive at the testing center early for any needed paperwork, to change your clothes, remove your jewelry, and to lock up your valuables. If you have any last minute questions, you should ask them before the test begins.

After telling you about the procedure, the MRI technician will have you lie on a thin mattress and will insert earplugs. In some testing centers, your head will be secured in one position with padding and a Velcro strap to prevent head movement. You will then be slid into a doughnut-shaped opening at one end of the MRI machine. This machine does not move, and its opening does not change in any way during the test. The technician will be outside the room you are in and will be in voice contact with you during the entire test. Usually, you will be able to see the technician through a window. Some machines have a mirror mounted above your head to allow you to see out at all times. Many MRI testing places are also able to play music during the test.

You will be instructed to be absolutely still while the machine is working. While working, it makes a banging noise the ear plugs are meant to protect against. Do not speak with the technician while the machine is making a noise unless an emergency arises.

Many times an MRI test includes the use of a chemical called gadolinium, which will help identify any abnormal brain growths. The chemical will either be injected directly into a vein, or an IV will be started to give the drug. You may experience a brief burning sensation in the area of the injection or infusion, but it will quickly pass, and the injection causes no other sensations.

You will be in the machine about 30 to 45 minutes. The banging noise will occur only part of the time.

An MRI may show some of the bony outer shell of the inner ear, such as in Figure C-5 but will not reveal the interior.

Insurance note: If you must get prior approval from your insurance company, make sure you have it before going for this test. If a test must be done in an "approved" facility, make sure the MRI testing center is included on your insurance company's list. Another word of caution: an MRI machine located within an approved hospital could be owned and operated by a separate group or business that is not approved. Ask.

On occasion, your doctor might suggest a magnetic resonance angiography (MRA) test. It evaluates blood flow in the area tested. Taking an MRA test will not seem any different from taking an MRI.

X-Rays

X-rays cannot diagnose BPPV. When X-rays are requested, they are used to look for abnormal growths or fractures or to view the anatomy around the ear(s).

Figure C-5: Magnetic resonance imaging (MRI) of the head. A cochlea and two semicircular canals are visible on the left.

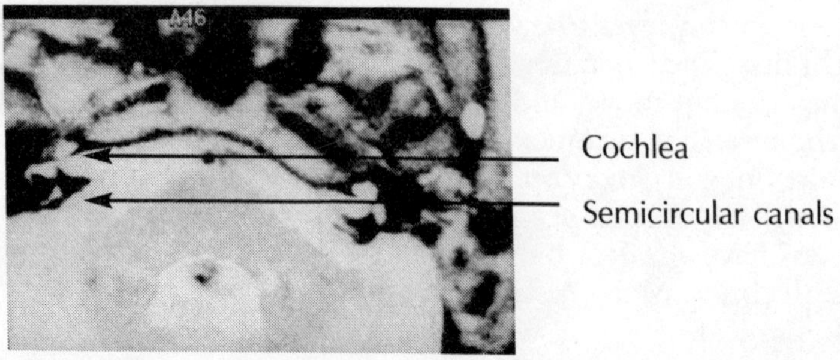

CT Scan

This type of X-ray series can find a fracture, erosion from a disease process, a congenital deformity, or demineralization of the bony labyrinth. Some doctors will arrange for a computerized tomography (CT) scan of the temporal bone before doing certain inner ear surgeries.

Blood Tests

No blood tests exist to detect the presence of BPPV. However, your doctor may order a battery of blood tests anyway. The tests are usually done to look for specific conditions known to cause some of the symptoms similar to those experienced with BPPV.

References

Baloh, R.W., Honrubia, V., and Jacobson, K. "Benign Positional Vertigo: Clinical and Oculogyric Features in 240 Cases." *Neurology*, 37:371-378, 1987.

Baloh, R.W., Yue, Q., Jacobson, K.M., and Honrubia, V. " Persistent Direction-Changing Positional Nystagmus: Another Variant of Benign Positional Nystagmus?" *Neurology*, 45:1297-1301, 1995.

Black, F.O., and Nashner, L.M. "Vestibulo-Spinal Control Differs in Patient with Reduced Versus Distorted Vestibular Function." *Acta Otolaryngologica Supp*, 406:110-114 1984.

Covera-Behar, G., Corvera, J., and Hernanadez, L.M. "Benign Positional Vertigo Produces a Specific Pattern of Abnormalities with High Frequency Vestibulo-Ocular Reflex Testing." *ENT Journal.* 73(10):768-771, 1994.

Dix, M.R., and Hallpike, C.S. "The Pathology, Symptomatology and Diagnosis of Certain Common Disorders of the Vestibular System." *Proceedings of the Royal Society of Medicine*, 45:341-354, 1952.

Fife, T.D. "Recognition and Management of Horizontal Canal Benign Positional Vertigo." *American Journal of Otology*, 19:345-351, 1998.

Furman, J.M., and Cass, S.P. *Balance Disorders: A Case-Study Approach*. Philadelphia: F.A. Davis, Company, 1996.

Gordon, N. "Post-Traumatic Vertigo with Special Reference to Positional Nystagmus." *The Lancet*, June 12, 1954.

Herdman, S.J. *Vestibular Rehabilitation*. Philadelphia: F.A. Davis Company, 1994.

Jacobson, G.P., Newman, C.W., and Kartush, J.M. *Handbook of Balance Function Testing*. San Diego: Singular Publishing Group, Inc., 1997.

Lanska, D.J., and Remler, B. "BPPV: Classic Descriptions, Origins of the Provocative Positioning Technique, and Conceptual Developments." *Neurology*, 48:1167-1177, 1997.

Mohr, D.N. "The Syndrome of Paroxysmal Positional Vertigo: A Review." *Western Journal of Medicine*, 145:645-650, 1986.

Norre, M. "Reliability of Examination Data in the Diagnosis of Benign Paroxysmal Positional Vertigo." *American Journal of Otology*, 16(6):806-810, 1995.

Nuti, D., Vannucchi, P., and Pagnini, P. "Benign Paroxysmal Positional Vertigo of the Horizontal Canal: A Form of Canalolithiasis with Variable Clinical Features." *Journal of Vestibular Research*, 6(3):173-184, 1996.

Schuknecht, H.F. "Cupulolithiasis." *Archives of Otolaryngology-Head and Neck Surgery*, 90:113-126, 1969.

Swartz, J.D., Daniels, D.L., Harnsberger, H.R., Shaffer, K.A., and Mark, L. "Balance and Equilibrium, I: The Vestibule and Semicircular Canals?" *American Journal of Neuroradiology*, 17:17-21, 1996.

Von Gierke, H.E., et al. "Evaluation of Tests for Vestibular Function." Aviation, Space and Environmental Medicine, A1-A34, 1992.

Appendix D: Drugs

General Drug Information

Drugs are almost never used to treat the milder forms of BPPV. The vertigo is too intense and too short in duration for drugs to affect it. Drugs are sometimes used in the more severe types of BPPV and in people with BPPV plus another vestibular problem.

If your doctor has prescribed drugs for you, respect their power. Drugs can be good in the right amount for the right condition, but they can also cause harm. Some bad results from drug therapy such as allergic reactions probably can't be prevented, but other bad results can be avoided by following some rules.

If you have allergic reactions to anything, wear a medic-alert kind of necklace or bracelet listing the substances you must avoid. (You can write to a company called MedicAlert at 2323 Colorado Ave., Turlock, CA 95382 for details or call them at 1-800-763-3428.) Also, you should mention the substances you must avoid to every health-care professional you visit as a patient. Never assume that the doctor or nurse or other health-care professional already knows about your allergies.

You should also wear a medic-alert kind of necklace or bracelet if you:

- are taking a drug that should not be stopped suddenly.
- are on a special diet.
- have a hearing loss.
- take a drug called an MAO inhibitor.
- have any serious problems such as heart, lung, liver, or kidney disease.
- have glaucoma.
- have an enlarged prostate.

When you get a prescription from your doctor, make sure you know:

- what the drug is. (See "Generic Names; Trade Names" later in this chapter.)
- what it is supposed to do.
- how to take it.
- how much to take.

- when to take it.
- what changes you should report to the doctor if they occur.
- what drugs and other substances it interacts with. (Most drugs, when combined with certain other drugs and substances, can cause effects different from the effects they cause by themselves.)

Make a list of all your medications (including generic and trade names), when you take them, how much you take, the name of the doctor who prescribed them, and how long you have been taking them. Keep a copy of the list at home and another with you at all times.

When you see your doctor(s), review your medication list with them or any other health care providers giving you prescriptions or treatments.

If you take more than one drug, make sure you are taking the right one at the right time for the right thing. Check the label each time to verify you have the correct one.

Store your drugs in a dark, dry place with a temperature between 59 and 86 degrees for pills and below 77 degrees for suppositories. **(Don't store them in your bathroom; the hot air and humidity can alter them.)**

Pills and suppositories can change in heat. Don't leave them in a car, particularly when the sun is out and the air temperature is warm.

When you have to take a pill (tablet, capsule, or caplet), take it with a full glass of water unless instructed otherwise. Also, when possible, sit up for a while after swallowing a pill to help it get to your stomach.

To avoid confusion and protect your medicine from light, keep your medicine in its original container.

If any of the instructions on the medication's label are changed later, note the change and the date of change on the label, or attach a separate note to the medicine container.

Get all of your drugs from the same pharmacy. Always ask if any new drugs you are planning to take are compatible with the older ones; this includes over-the-counter medications and any other drugs you are taking. (If you get drugs from several places, the pharmacists will not know all the drugs you are taking and cannot automatically check for possible drug conflicts.)

Don't crush pills or open capsules unless you have been told it is OK for that particular medicine. The pill's packaging can affect where and how the contents are released into your body.

If you have small children living with you or visiting, be careful where you store your medicines, and use childproof caps. If you visit someone with small children, keep your medications where the children can't find them.

If you think there is a problem with any of your medications or that you are having a problem caused by them, tell your doctor(s) and keep on telling them until you feel your concerns have been heard and addressed. If you believe a medicine is causing a problem and a specialist has not listened to your concerns, try seeing your primary care doctor (family doctor) and discussing the situation with him or her. You can also discuss your medications and problems with your pharmacist and ask her or him to talk to your doctor.

Getting Drug Information

You can get reliable drug information from the doctor prescribing it or from the pharmacist dispensing it.

Bookstores and/or libraries have many excellent drug guides written for the public.

People who want more in-depth information can look through a nursing pharmacology textbook; these usually explain pertinent structure and function and are written for nursing students just out of high school. Many community colleges offer nursing courses, and their textbooks should be available in the school's library.

If you want even more information, you can try a pharmacology book like Goodman and Gilman's *The Pharmacological Basis of Therapeutics* or Katzung's *Basic and Clinical Pharmacology*, written for doctors, or Hansten and Horn's *Drug Interactions: Analysis and Management*. Texts like these assume that the reader has a solid grasp of medical terminology, and anatomy and physiology.

Generic Names; Trade Names

Drugs often have two different names, *generic* and *trade*. The generic name for a medicine is the one all drug companies can use to refer to a medication because the name is not owned by anyone. It might be considered the more "scientific" name and the one more difficult to pronounce, spell, and remember. When you choose a generic drug, you will probably get a brand made by a company other than the company that first marketed the drug.

The trade name is a medication name owned by a specific company. Trade names are usually shorter and easier to spell and remember than the generic drug names. Sometimes the name describes the use of the drug in some way. One popular inner ear drug, meclizine (generic name), is called Antivert (trade name) by the company that sells it.

Throughout this book, drugs are referred to in a standard manner. The first letter in the generic name, as in meclizine, is lowercase (unless appearing as the first letter in a sentence), and the first letter in a trade name is uppercase, as in Antivert.

Symptom Blocking Drugs

The best drug treatment is one that prevents or eliminates a problem. Unfortunately, no such drug exists for BPPV. No available drugs can prevent BPPV from occurring in the first place or stop it once it has started, nor are any available drugs capable of dissolving the canal debris in order to stop the episodes of vertigo.

> "No medication worked, and, believe me, I tried everything from anti-nauseants to decongestants."
>
> —D. H., letter to the author, 1998

Drugs may be used as pre-medication before canalith repositioning. In certain circumstances, drugs may also be used in some people with BPPV to control any of the following:

- symptoms created by an accompanying vestibular problem such as Meniere's disease
- nausea, dizziness, and/or motion sickness occurring between episodes of positional vertigo
- motion sickness during a trip
- anxiety, on occasion

Symptom-blocking drugs are grouped into four categories in this chapter, as follows:

- motion-sickness drugs: meclizine (Antivert, etc.), dimenhydrinate (Dramamine Original Formula), diphenhydramine (Benadryl, etc.), and scopolamine
- drugs used for nausea and vomiting: promethazine (Phenergan) and prochlorperazine (Compazine, etc.)
- anti-anxiety/anti-vertigo drugs: diazepam (Valium), alprazolam (Xanax), lorazepam (Ativan), and clonazepam (Klonopin)
- alternative drugs (Vertigoheel)

Although these drugs belong to different groups and work in different ways, similarities exist, as follows:

- They should not be used with alcohol, barbiturates, tranquilizers, sleeping medicine, allergy medicines, anesthetics, pain medications, sedatives, antidepressants, marijuana or other street drugs, or with each other unless under the direction of a physician. Any drug that causes depression of the brain will also increase their effect and can cause great drowsiness.
- Many of these drugs can cause a dry mouth. For this problem, try rinsing your mouth, drinking fluids, sucking on ice or sugar-free hard candy, or taking a saliva substitute such as Moi-Stir, or Xero-Lube. If you experience a dry mouth much of the time, see your

dentist; a dry mouth can increase the likelihood of tooth decay and gum disease.

- Drowsiness is common with many of these drugs. You should not drive or do anything else requiring coordination and thorough thought if you are experiencing drowsiness. Do not drive if your vision is blurry.
- Many of these drugs are antihistamines. If you are taking an antihistamine and are sent for allergy testing, remind your primary doctor that you are taking it since it may interfere with the testing. Also, inform the allergist that you are taking the drug.

In this appendix, we have included more information on drugs that are available over-the-counter than on drugs available by prescription only since people taking the over-the-counter variety may not have as much information from other sources. More information about all of the drugs in this chapter (and other drugs sometimes used to treat the symptoms of BPPV) is available from your physician and your pharmacist.

Motion Sickness Drugs

Special note: If you develop eye pain, see halos around lights, or develop blurred vision (all symptoms of glaucoma) while taking any of the motion sickness drugs, report it to your doctor.

Meclizine

Also known as: **Antivert, Bonine, Dramamine Less Drowsy Formula.**

Meclizine is an over-the-counter antihistamine used to decrease or stop nausea, vomiting, and the dizziness of motion sickness. It acts directly on the inner ear, is able to decrease the amount of vestibular information the brain receives, and acts on the area of the brain responsible for nausea and vomiting.

Meclizine begins to work 30 to 60 minutes after you take it. Its peak of action occurs in one to two hours and continues for eight to 24 hours.

Meclizine can also be obtained with a prescription. Check with your pharmacist to determine the least expensive product you can buy. A prescription from your doctor may be less expensive than buying an over-the-counter product.

Limits

Not everyone can use meclizine. People with asthma, glaucoma, emphysema, prostate enlargement, heart failure, intestinal blockage, heart rhythm problems, liver disease, urinary tract blockage, pulmonary (lung) disease, someone missing substantial vestibular function in both ears, and/or someone who is pregnant may be told by their doctors not to take this drug.

If you are asked to take this drug regularly, you can expect the drowsiness to decrease, maybe even disappear.

Dimenhydrinate

Also known as: **Dramamine Original Formula. In Canada, Gravol.**

Dimenhydrinate is an over-the-counter antihistamine used to decrease or stop nausea and vomiting and the dizziness of motion sickness. It begins to work 15 to 30 minutes after you swallow it and lasts four to six hours.

Limits

If you have prostate problems, glaucoma, urinary tract blockage or difficulty urinating, asthma, heart rhythm problems, convulsive disorders, stomach ulcers and/or significant bilateral vestibular losses, you may be told by your doctor not to take dimenhydrinate.

If you are instructed to take this drug on a daily schedule, the drowsiness can be expected to decrease, maybe even disappear.

Diphenhydramine

Also known as: **Benadryl.**

Diphenhydramine is another over-the-counter antihistamine used to decrease or stop nausea, vomiting, and the dizziness of motion sickness. It begins to work in 60 minutes, hits peak action in two to four hours, and lasts four to seven hours.

Limits

People with acute asthma, glaucoma, stomach ulcer, peptic ulcer, urinary tract obstruction, hyperthyroidism, gastrointestinal (GI) obstruction or stenosis (narrowing), convulsive disorders, cardiovascular disease, diabetes mellitus, thyroid disease, heart disease, asthma, epilepsy and/or pregnant women may be told by their doctors not to take the drug.

If you are instructed to take this drug on a daily schedule, the drowsiness can be expected to decrease, maybe even disappear.

Scopolamine

Also known as: **Transderm-Scop. In Canada, Transderm-V.**

Scopolamine, the only drug in this group that is not an antihistamine, is available by prescription to prevent the nausea and vomiting of motion sickness. It usually does not affect the violent positional vertigo of BPPV. The patch is designed to deliver medication for three days; the best effects are not available until the patch has been in place for as long as 12 hours.

Cautions

- Do not rub your eyes after applying or removing the scopolamine patch unless you have washed your hands.
- Be careful not to get overheated while taking this drug since it may decrease your ability to sweat. Exercise, hot weather, hot tubs, saunas, etc., could cause you to become lightheaded.

Warning

Most doctors do not prescribe scopolamine for use on a regular basis (such as daily for weeks or months) for BPPV because many people go through a withdrawal period when stopping the drug. Withdrawal symptoms can include dizziness, nausea, vomiting, headache, disturbance of equilibrium, return of vertigo, anxiety, irritability, nightmares, and trouble sleeping. Tolerance to the drug may also occur; that is, the same amount of the drug may no longer bring about the same amount of relief.

Drugs Used for Nausea, Vomiting

The medications most commonly prescribed to prevent or stop nausea and vomiting associated with vestibular symptoms are described in this section.

Promethazine

Also known as: **Phenergan.**

Promethazine is both an antihistamine and phenothiazine derivative available only by prescription. It is used for sedation and to stop nausea and vomiting caused by motion sickness or other factors. It is available for home use as a tablet, oral solution, and as a rectal suppository, and it works within 20 minutes.

Suppositories should be stored in a refrigerator between 36 and 46 degrees Fahrenheit.

Prochlorperazine

Also known as: **Compazine, Stemetil.**

Prochlorperazine, a prescription medicine, is used for its anti-nausea and anti-vomiting properties. It is not thought to be effective in preventing vertigo or motion sickness. It is available for home use as a tablet, oral solution, extended-release capsule, and rectal suppository. The suppository works within 60 minutes, and the tablets/caplets work within 30 to 40 minutes.

This drug can cause side effects called an extrapyramidal reaction.

In depth: Extrapyramidal reactions or symptoms are side effects that can occur when a drug affects certain areas of the brain. Extrapyramidal reactions can be grouped into three types: acute dystonic reactions, akathisia, and Parkinsonism.

Acute dystonic reactions may include neck muscle or back spasms, mandibular tics (jaw jerking), and difficulty talking. These reactions usually occur within 24 to 48 hours of starting drug therapy or when there is an increase in drug dose.

Motor restlessness or akathisia includes agitation, jitteriness, inability to sit still, tapping of the feet, or a strong urge to move around. In most cases akathisia occurs within two to three days of therapy, although it can occur later (up to several weeks).

Parkinsonism appears as a mask-like face, drooling, tremors, pill-rolling motion of the fingers, and/or a shuffling gait (walk).

In addition to extrapyramidal reactions, a dyskinesia (tardive dyskinesia) or difficulty in performing voluntary movements can occur. Tardive dyskinesia appears as rhythmic, involuntary movements of the tongue, face, mouth, or jaw. It may occur after long term administration of agents like prochlorperazine, or after a certain cumulative (total) dose is reached.

Anti-Anxiety Drugs

The anti-anxiety drugs described in this section are all known as benzodiazepines. They act in the brain to produce their effects. As anti-anxiety drugs they decrease anxiety, have a calming effect, and can cause drowsiness and sleep. These drugs also function as vestibular suppressants. They are able to help cover up vertigo in some cases; however, the vertigo of BPPV is not generally present long enough to be treated by these drugs. These drugs also have muscle relaxant effects. They are all prescription drugs and have the ability to cause addiction.

None should be stopped abruptly if it has been taken routinely daily for four to six weeks or longer. Withdrawal symptoms can occur when these drugs are stopped abruptly or if the dose is severely reduced. These drugs stay in the body for days after the drug is stopped, so withdrawal symptoms may not occur until a few days later.

Diazepam

Also known as: **Valium.**

Diazepam is used to decrease anxiety, decrease muscle tension, and to cover up vestibular symptoms. Its effects can be felt in 30 minutes.

In depth (withdrawal): Withdrawal symptoms can include tremor, difficulty concentrating, anxiety, agitation, increased sensitivity to light and sound, strange sensations, numbness/tingling, muscle jerking, sleep disturbances, depersonalization, abnormal perception of movement, dizziness, abdominal and muscle cramps, vomiting, sweating, and convulsions. The symptoms of withdrawal may seem more like a return of the original symptoms than a reaction to stopping the drug.

Alprazolam

Also known as: **Xanax.**

Alprazolam is used to decrease anxiety and to cover up vestibular symptoms. The pill form begins to work within one to two hours.

Special warning: Some people have confused Xanax with Zantac, a stomach medication available by prescription and over-the-counter. Double-check your medicine before taking it, particularly if you are taking a large number of drugs.

Avoid drinking grapefruit juice within several hours of taking alprazolam, since the combination may result in significant enhanced effects of the alprazolam. (Enhanced means it will become stronger then intended by the prescribing physician.)

Withdrawal symptoms can include heightened sensory perception, impaired concentration, muscle cramps, decreased appetite, weight loss, muscle twitch, diarrhea, blurred vision, and numbness or a tingling sensation.

When alprazolam is used to treat panic disorder, stopping the drug can cause a "rebound" of the symptoms, a reappearance of panic at or above the level previously experienced.

Lorazepam

Also known as: **Ativan.**

Lorazepam is used to decrease anxiety and vestibular symptoms. Besides being available in tablet form, it is also available as a sublingual tablet that can be placed under the tongue, from where it is absorbed into the blood stream. The peak effect of lorazepam usually occurs in two hours.

Clonazepam

Also known as: **Klonopin.**

Clonazepam is used to decrease vestibular symptoms. It begins to work within one hour with its peak action occurring in one to two hours.

Alternative Drugs

Vertigoheel

Vertigoheel is a homeopathic combination remedy made from botanical, zoological, and mineral ingredients. It is prescribed by homeopathic physicians for use in vertigo, related imbalance disorders, and in the prevention or treatment of motion sickness. How it works is not fully understood, but it is thought to cause stimulation in some areas of the brain.

References

_____. *Consumer Guide to Prescription Drugs*. Illinois: Publications International, Ltd., 1995.

_____. *Drug Information for the Health Care Professional.* Rockville: United States Pharmacopeial Convention, 1990.

_____. *Physicians' Desk Reference*. Oradell, N.J.: Medical Economics, 1998.

_____. *Physicians' Desk Reference*. Oradell, N.J.: Medical Economics, 1999.

_____. *The PDR Family Guide to Prescription Drugs*. Montvale, N.J.: Medical Economics, 1995.

Baloh, R.W., and Halmagyi, V.G. *Clinical Neurophysiology*. Second edition. Philadelphia: F.A. Davis Company, 1990.

Baloh, R.W., and Halmagyi, V.G. *Disorders of the Vestibular System*. New York: Oxford University Press, 1996.

Fujino, A., Tokumasu, K., *et al.* "Vestibular Training for Acute Unilateral Vestibular Disturbances: Its Efficacy in Comparison with Antivertigo Drugs." *Acta Otolaryngologica Suppl (Stockh)*, 524:21-26, 1996.

Furman, J.M., and Cass, S.P. *Balance Disorders: A Case-Study Approach*. Philadelphia: F.A. Davis Company, 1996.

Griffith, H.W. *Complete Guide to Prescription and Non-Prescription Drugs*. Sixth edition. The Body Press, 1989.

Hain, T.C. "Medical Treatment of Vertigo." *Vestibular Update*, 11:1-7, 1993.

Hardman, J.G., Gilman, A.G., and Limbird. L.E. *Goodman and Gilman's: The Pharmacological Basis of Therapeutics*. Ninth edition. New York: McGraw-Hill, 1996.

Katzung, B.G. *Basic and Clinical Pharmacology*. Sixth edition. Norwalk, Connecticut: Appleton and Lange, 1995.

Long, J.W., and Rybacki, J.J. *The Essential Guide to Prescription Drugs*. New York: Harper Perennial, 1994.

Norris, C.H. "Drugs Affecting the Inner Ear: A Review of Their Clinical Efficacy, Mechanisms of Action, Toxicity, and Place in Therapy." *Drugs*, 36:754-772, 1988.

Rowland, L.P. Merritt's *Textbook of Neurology*. Ninth edition. Pennsylvania: Williams and Wilkins, 1995.

Silverman, H.M. *The Pill Book*. Seventh edition. New York: Bantam Books, 1996.

Wilson, B.A., Shannon, M.T., and Stang, C.L. *Nurses' Drug Guide 1993*. Norwalk: Appleton and Lange, 1993.

Appendix E:

More Coping Tips

If you have a more severe form of BPPV; that is, if it has been present for a long time despite treatment, or if it is fairly constant, or if another vestibular problem is also present, coping can be a big, ongoing, and stressful activity. Here are additional coping tips, beyond those to be found in Chapter 12.

General Tips

Remove or firmly attach throw rugs to the floor. Limit clutter. Be careful when you walk on anything slippery such as snow, ice, or a wet surface. Have adequate lighting anyplace you go at night. Install nightlights. A cane or walking stick can help someone with particularly poor balance function.

> "Hold onto objects for support as needed, turn a light on when getting out of bed at night, be particularly careful getting in and out of the bathtub, but otherwise carry on with your daily routine if you can."
>
> —G. Hughes, M.D., *American Journal of Otology*, 1999

Fatigue

To prevent or relieve fatigue:

- Go at a slower pace if having bouts of vertigo.
- Get help when you need it.
- Because stress can lead to fatigue, reduce unproductive stress as much as possible. (See "Stress Control" later in this appendix.)
- Allow yourself enough time to get adequate sleep at night; you may need to make this a priority.
- Eat a well-balanced and adequate diet.
- Exercise regularly.
- Depression can lead to fatigue. If you think you might be depressed, get help from your primary care physician or a mental health professional.

Muscle and Joint Tightness or Pain

To prevent or relieve muscle and joint tightness or pain, get adequate exercise. (However, always check with your personal physician before undertaking an exercise program.)

Stress reduction and relaxation methods might also be beneficial, particularly if stress from anxiety is causing the tightness or pain.

Staggering

If you stagger or have difficulty walking straight:

- Use cues from your surroundings about the location of horizontal and vertical.
- Walk along a wall rather than in the open.
- Wear flat shoes with non-skid soles.
- Pick something in the distance to walk towards.

Bothersome Bright Lights

While you are outdoors, wear sunglasses that block glare. Use a sun hat, sun visor, or baseball cap to supplement the sunglasses.

Poor Depth Perception

On an overcast day, try wearing glasses that are yellow or amber.

Reading

- Use a non-flickering light source. Don't try to read with a fluorescent light or from the light generated by your TV or computer monitor.
- Move from word to word by placing your finger under each word to help keep your eyes on the right spot.
- Place a ruler (a solid ruler, not one you can see through) under the sentence you are trying to read.
- Read in a place that is quiet and visually calm.

Poor Memory

To help compensate for memory problems, make notes about things you want to remember, or use a tape recorder. Use "cheat" sheets when appropriate.

Difficulty Writing

To adjust to writing difficulty, work on important things when you are rested and without distractions. If what you are writing is really important, find someone to proofread it for you.

Persistent Symptoms

To deal with chronic problems:

- Take one day at a time.
- Avoid the aggravating positions as needed.
- Don't sleep on the affected ear.
- Try sleeping with your head elevated by a couple of pillows.
- Ask your doctor about anti-vertigo or anti-vomiting medications useful during long car trips or other activities known to cause you problems.
- Get a physician you can work with and who is not frustrated by the chronic nature of your case.

> "I spent six months sleeping sitting up on the couch because lying too flat made it worse. I've learned to sleep on three pillows."
>
> —B.C., New York, letter to the author, 1999

Stress Control

Many articles, videotapes, audiotapes, and books discuss stress, how to use it, or how to lessen it. The three-step approach to stress, outlined below, is just one of many:

- Recognize your symptoms of stress. Tune in to your body; listen to what it is telling you. Do you have warning signals? Does your head ache? Do you feel tension in the back of your neck? By heeding these signals, you can recognize that stress is beginning to affect you.
- Identify the sources of your stress. Sometimes you can handle big problems more easily than everyday ones. Worrying about little things wastes lots of energy.
- Take action. What can you do to change? Promote your health by eating better, by getting adequate rest and exercise, and by following medical advice. Cut down on the unnecessary, and do the most important things first. Being actively involved with a support group may be helpful. Don't be afraid to reach out for help.

Your personal philosophy of life and your spirituality can make a difference. If you practice a religion, you might find prayer a comfort.

Openly communicate with friends. Learn to laugh. A sense of humor is an excellent coping mechanism. Take responsibility for the stress in your life.

> "I am looking forward to my miracle healing that I know will come some day, and thank God for the little breaks now and again."
>
> —B.C., New York, letter to the author, 1999

Advice and tips are available from many sources for making life with BPPV easier. By picking and choosing appropriately, you may be able to improve your life.

Drug Effects

The drugs used on occasion to reduce symptoms in more extreme cases of BPPV can cause a number of side effects, many of which could affect safety. Blurred vision, sleepiness, slowed reaction times, diminished balance ability, and slow decision-making can create danger in many activities such as taking a shower, slicing food in the kitchen, cutting wood with a chain saw, operating power tools, driving a car, and anything else that requires alertness and hand-eye coordination. When starting a new drug, don't drive until you know how it affects you.

Some evidence indicates that people over 65 years old who are taking anti-anxiety drugs have a 45 percent higher rate of traffic accidents during the first week they take the drugs and a 25 percent higher rate overall than do people over 65 years who are not taking the drugs. Other evidence suggests that seniors on antidepressants have an increased chance of being in an automobile accident. And other research suggests that people age 55 and older taking a benzodiazepine (Valium, Xanax, Ativan) have a larger chance of falling and breaking a thigh bone than people not taking one of these drugs.

Many times drug-related symptoms abate over time as the body adjusts to the presence of the drug(s). When first starting any course of drug treatment, be particularly careful in all your activities, particularly driving, until you learn how the drug affects you.

Regaining Self-Confidence

- Take control as best you can.
- Prepare for any situation you can predict.
- Learn all about your disease and the treatment you are undergoing.
- Be involved in your care.

- Set your own goals. Don't automatically adopt those of your peers or of society.
- Determine your priorities.
- When you are able, look for the positives in your life.

More on Driving

Skills and Physical Abilities

Driving is a complex activity requiring both mental and physical abilities. According to the American Automobile Association, safe and efficient driving depends upon:

- accurately identifying elements of the traffic scene
- making a correct interpretation of the traffic scene
- making the proper response

In other words vision, thought and physical ability, including strength, flexibility, and coordination, are needed to drive safely. As much as 90 percent of driving depends upon vision. Driving also requires the ability to think, to understand what is being seen, and to act upon it. According to the American Automobile Association, drivers must make 20 decisions per mile during routine driving and as many as 200 per mile during city driving. The faster you drive, the faster you must be able to carry out the tasks.

Many symptoms from both the ear and from anti-vertigo drugs can impair the ability to drive. These symptoms include positional vertigo, blurred vision, bouncing vision, sleepiness/fatigue, slowed reaction time, visually stimulated disorientation, stiff neck and/or mental distraction, and distortion of lights, such as headlights, in darkness.

The National Commission on Sleep disorders estimates that 42 to 54 percent of all accidents are related to drowsiness and that drowsiness causes 36 percent of all fatal accidents.

No studies have been published about people distracted by vestibular sensations while driving, but one study revealed a connection between another kind of distraction and car wrecks. The study found that people who use cell phones while driving have a quadrupled chance of having an accident. (This statistic held true even for drivers using cell phones not held to the ear by hand.)

To Drive or Not

When thinking about your fitness to drive, put safety ahead of need or desire and think about the following quote from the

American Automobile Association, "Driving in today's fast-paced world is difficult enough without the additional hindrance of dizziness, blurred vision, or drowsiness."

Don't drive if you have:

- blurred vision
- difficulty thinking, remembering or making decisions
- a stiff neck that prevents observing your total environment when behind the wheel
- positional vertigo from any head position or movement necessary to drive
- visually stimulated vertigo or spatial disorientation

If you feel too sick or tired to drive, don't do it. If you can't see properly or make rapid decisions, don't get behind the wheel. Get a lift from a friend or neighbor, use public transportation, or take a taxi instead.

References

_____. American Automobile Association. "Alcohol, Vision, and Driving" (Traffic Safety Department brochure #3385), 1975.

_____. American Automobile Association. "Straight Talk for Older Adults: Good Vision Vital to Good Driving" (Corporate Communications brochure #2286), 1992.

_____. American Automobile Association. "Straight Talk for Older Drivers: Rx for Safe Driving" (Corporate Communications brochure #2288), 1993.

Galski, T., Ehle, H.T., and Williams, J.B. "Estimates of Driving Abilities and Skills in Different Conditions." *American Journal of Occupational Therapy*, 52(4):268-274, 1998.

Hemmelgarn, B., et al. "Benzodiazepine Use and the Risk of Motor Vehicle Crash in the Elderly." *Journal of the American Medical Association*, 278:27-31, 1997.

Herings, R.M., et al. "Benzodiazepines and the Risk of Falling Leading to Femur Factures: Dosage More Important Than Elimination Half-Life." *Archives of Internal Medicine*, 155(16):1801-1807, 1995.

Leveille, S.G., et al. "Psychoactive Medications and Injurious Motor Vehicle Collisions Involving Older Drivers." *Epidemiology*, 5(6):591-598, 1994.

McCloskey, L.W., Koepsell, T.D., Wolf, M.E., and Buchner, D.M. "Motor Vehicle Collision Injuries and Sensory Impairments of Older Drivers. *Ageing*, 23(4):267-273, 1994.

Parnes, L.S., and Sindwani, R. "Impact of Vestibular Disorders on Fitness to Drive: A Census of the American Neurotology Society." *American Journal of Otology*, 18:79-85, 1997.

Redelmeier, D.A., and Tibshirani, R.J. "Association Between Cellular Telephone Calls and Motor Vehicle Collisions." *New England Journal of Medicine*, 336(7):453-458, 1997.

Sindwani, R., Parnes, L.S., Goebel, J.A., and Cass, S.P. "Approach to the Vestibular Patient and Driving: A Patient Perspective." *Otolaryngology-Head and Neck Surgery*, 121:12-17, 1999.

Sindwani, R., and Parnes, L.S. "Reporting of Vestibular Patients Who Are Unfit to Drive: Survey of Canadian Otolaryngologists." *Journal of Otolaryngology*, 26(2):104-111, 1997.

Teran-Santos, J., Jimenez-Gomez, A., and Cordero-Guevara, J. "The Association Between Sleep Apnea and the Risk of Traffic Accidents." *New England Journal of Medicine*, 340(11):847-851, 1999.

Glossary

The following glossary briefly defines some of the terms used in this book. You can best understand these and many other terms in the context of the chapters in which they appear or by reviewing anatomical illustrations. For example, for definitions of surgical terms see Chapter 10, "Surgery," and for definitions of professional specialties see Chapter 13, "Who's Who in Otologic Health Care." To find the exact places in this book where certain terms are used, please refer to the Index.

Ampulla. The bulbous end of a semicircular canal.

Anterior. Front.

Antihistamine. A drug used to relieve the symptoms of allergies. On occasion, an antihistamine can also be used to treat vertigo and the nausea and vomiting related to it.

Ataxia. Lack of coordination.

Audiogram. The "standard" hearing test that usually includes pure tones and speech.

Auditory. Refers to the sense of hearing.

Aural. Pertaining to the ear.

Auricle. The outside flap of the ear. Also called the *pinna*.

Balance. A state of repose between two or more antagonistic forces that exactly counteract each other. With relation to human balance, this generally means using your muscles to counteract gravity and other forces by keeping your center of gravity aligned over your feet.

Benign Paroxysmal Positional Vertigo (BPPV). Syndrome or disorder involving episodes of vertigo occurring with particular head movements. Sometimes also called BPV (benign positional vertigo) or BPPN (benign paroxysmal positional nystagmus).

Brain stem. The part of the brain that performs motor, sensory, and reflex functions.

Caloric test. A test that requires irrigation of the ear canal with warm and/or cool water or air to measure vestibular functions.

Canalith. Calcium carbonate crystal present in a semicircular canal.

Canalithiasis. Condition involving debris ("ear rocks") free-floating in a semicircular canal.

Center of gravity. That point in a thing around which its weight is evenly distributed or balanced. Point of equilibrium.

Central nervous system. The brain and spinal cord.

Cerebellum. The part of the brain responsible for coordination.

Cerumen. Ear wax.

Cilia. Hairlike projections on the surfaces of some cells.

Cochlea. The end organ of hearing.

Computerized tomography (CT or CAT) scan. A scan using computers and X-rays to obtain highly detailed, three-dimensional information about body tissues and bone.

Cupula. Gelatinous mass covering the hair cells in the ampulla of a semicircular canal.

Cupulolithiasis. Condition involving debris ("ear rocks") adhering to a cupula of a semicircular canal.

Degeneration. Deterioration or impairment.

Disequilibrium. Vague sense of unsteadiness, imbalance, tilting, or bumping into things that can occur in association with vestibular problems.

Dix-Hallpike test. Maneuver to see if nystagmus occurs during certain changes in head position. The test is useful in diagnosing BPPV.

Ear drum. Common name for tympanic membrane. It forms the boundary between the outer and middle ears.

Ear "rocks." See **Otoliths**.

Electrocochleography (EcoG). Computerized test measuring the way a specific sound moves electrically through the cochlea and the ear end of the vestibulo-cochlear nerve (at the beginning of its trip to the brain).

Electronystagmography (ENG). A method of measuring eye movements. A battery of ENG tests, including the caloric ENG, may be used to assess relationships between the eyes and the vestibular system and help diagnose the cause of dizziness or vertigo.

Endolymph. Fluid within the membranous labyrinth of the inner ear.

Endolymphatic hydrops. Excessive amount of endolymph. Increased pressure from this endolymph can damage any part of the vestibular apparatus or the cochlea.

Equilibrium. State of repose between two or more antagonistic forces that exactly counteract each other. With relation to human balance this generally means using your muscles to counteract gravity and other forces by keeping your center of gravity aligned over your feet.

Etiology. Science and study of the causes of disease and their mode of operation.

Eustachian tube. Hourglass-shaped tube connecting the middle ear with the area of the throat behind the nose.

Fistula. Abnormal opening from one internal organ to another or leading to a surface. Fistulas can occur between the inner ear and the middle ear.

Frenzel glasses. Goggles or lenses that magnify your eyes and prevent you from fixing your vision on an external object. This makes it easier for an examiner to observe your eyes for movement abnormalities.

Gait. Manner of walking.

Giddiness. Dizziness, lightheadedness.

Hair cell. Cylindrical inner ear cell with cilia (hairlike projections) protruding from one end. When vestibular hair cells in the utricle, saccule, or semicircular canals are stimulated by head movements, they secrete a chemical (neurotransmitter) that starts an electrical signal on its way to the brain via the nervous system.

Hallpike test. See **Dix-Hallpike test**.

Hyperacusis. Abnormal sensitivity to sound. It does not usually include vertigo caused by sound.

Hyperactive. More active than normal.

Hypoactive. Less active than normal.

Idiopathic. Of unknown cause.

Incus. One of three middle ear bones. Also called the *anvil*, it lies between the malleus and the stapes.

Inner ear. Fluid-filled system of chambers and passageways encased in the temporal bone. The inner ear includes the end organs of hearing and balance and is also called the *labyrinth*.

Labyrinth. Complex series of chambers and passageways of the inner ear, including the hearing and balance parts.

Labyrinthitis. Inflammation of the labyrinth or part of it.

Lateral. On the side.

Macula. In the inner ear, a tiny area of neural tissue in the saccule or utricle.

Magnetic resonance imaging (MRI). Diagnostic tool that produces cross-sectional images of parts of the body. An MRI of the brain can reveal the presence of tumors, stroke damage, and some other abnormalities.

Malleus. Outermost of the three ossicles (middle-ear bones). It is sometimes called the hammer.

Mastoid. Bone, partly filled with air spaces, located behind the ear.

Meniere's disease. Inner ear disorder of unknown cause characterized by distinct spontaneous episodes of vertigo lasting minutes to hours, hearing loss, and ear ringing and/or ear pressure.

Middle ear. Part of the ear that reaches from the ear drum to the outer surfaces of the oval and round windows.

Motion intolerance. Strong symptoms such as vertigo or nausea arising from head movement. These symptoms may cause avoidance of movement.

Neurotransmitter. Chemical that carries a nerve signal.

Nystagmus. Abnormal eye jerking.

Oscillopsia. Visual illusion that stationary objects are bobbing to and fro, back and forth, or up and down.

Ossicles. The three tiny bones of the middle ear.

Otic capsule. Outer shell of the bony labyrinth.

Otoliths. Crystalline particles of calcium carbonate and a protein adhering to the gelatinous membrane of the maculae of the utricle and saccule. Sometimes called "ear rocks."

Otoconia. Otoliths.

Otolithic membrane. Gelatinous-like material resting on the hair cells of the utricle or saccule.

Oval window. One of two covered openings between the middle ear and the inner ear.

Perilymph. Fluid surrounding and cushioning the membranous labyrinth.

Pinna. External, visible part of the ear. Also called the *auricle*.

Posterior. Back.

Proprioception. Gathering information via sensors in muscles, tendons, joints, ligaments, and connective tissue. The information is about gravity, body position, external surfaces, and the length and motion of the muscles and joints.

Round window. Membrane-covered opening between the inner ear and the middle ear.

Saccule. Inner ear chamber containing hair cells that sense gravity as well as movement in a straight line.

Semicircular canal. Curved inner ear structure, filled with endolymph, ending in a cupula with hair cells that sense angular head movement in the plane of the canal. Each inner ear has three semicircular canals; each canal is roughly perpendicular to the other two.

Sixth sense. The sense of balance.

Spatial disorientation. Confusion about one's position in space. This might include confusion about the location of vertical and horizontal

Spinal tap. Removal of fluid from the spinal column in order to reveal information about the spinal cord and brain. Also called *lumbar puncture*.

Stapes. The innermost of the three middle-ear bones. It is sometimes referred to as the *stirrup* because of its shape.

Syndrome. All of the signs and symptoms of a disease process taken together and constituting the picture of the disease.

Temporal bone. The part of the skull in which the inner ear is located.

Tinnitus. Hissing, ringing, or other abnormal noises in the ears. Commonly called "ringing in the ears."

Tympanic membrane. Ear drum.

Unilateral. Involving only one ear.

Utricle. Inner ear chamber containing hair cells responsible for sensing movement in a straight line and gravity.

Vertigo. Perception of movement (either of yourself or of objects around you) that is not occurring or is occurring differently from what you perceive.

Vestibular. Related to the balance parts of the inner ear and related structures.

Vestibular ocular reflex (VOR). Involuntary eye movements caused by stimulating the vestibular system.

Vestibulo-cochlear nerve. Nerve from the brain that is essential to the senses of hearing and balance. Also called *eighth cranial nerve*, *auditory nerve*, or *acoustic nerve*.

Index

Bold page numbers refer to definitions; italic page numbers refer to illustrations.

C

Bold page numbers refer to definitions; italic page numbers refer to illustrations.

D

Bold page numbers refer to definitions; italic page numbers refer to illustrations.

Bold page numbers refer to definitions; italic page numbers refer to illustrations.

Bold page numbers refer to definitions; italic page numbers refer to illustrations.

J

K

L

M

Bold page numbers refer to definitions; italic page numbers refer to illustrations.

Bold page numbers refer to definitions; italic page numbers refer to illustrations.

Bold page numbers refer to definitions; italic page numbers refer to illustrations.

R

S

Bold page numbers refer to definitions; italic page numbers refer to illustrations.

T

U

Bold page numbers refer to definitions; italic page numbers refer to illustrations.